CALCULUS DISEASE

Other titles in the *New Clinical Applications* Series:

Dermatology (Series Editor Dr J. L. Verbov)
Dermatological Surgery
Superficial Fungal Infections
Talking Points in Dermatology – I
Treatment in Dermatology
Current Concepts in Contact Dermatitis
Talking Points in Dermatology – II

Cardiology (Series Editor Dr D. Longmore)
Cardiology Screening

Rheumatology (Series Editors Dr J. J. Calabro and Dr W. Carson Dick)
Ankylosing Spondylitis
Infections and Arthritis

Nephrology (Series Editor Dr G. R. D. Catto)
Continuous Ambulatory Peritoneal Dialysis
Management of Renal Hypertension
Chronic Renal Failure
Calculus Disease
Pregnancy and Renal Disorders
Multisystem Diseases
Glomerulonephritis I
Glomerulonephritis II

NEW CLINICAL APPLICATIONS NEPHROLOGY

CALCULUS DISEASE

Editor

G. R. D. CATTO
MD, FRCP, FRCP(G)

Reader in Medicine
University of Aberdeen
UK

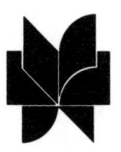

KLUWER ACADEMIC PUBLISHERS

DORDRECHT · BOSTON · LONDON

Distributors

for the United States and Canada: Kluwer Academic Publishers, PO Box 358, Accord Station, Hingham, MA 02018-0358, USA
for all other countries: Kluwer Academic Publishers Group, Distribution Center, PO Box 322, 3300 AH Dordrecht, The Netherlands

British Library Cataloguing in Publication Data

Calculus disease.
  1. Man. Kidneys. Calculi
  I. Catto, Graeme R. D. (Graeme Robertson Dawson), *1945–*   II. Series
  616.6'22

  ISBN 0–7462–0074–9
  ISBN 0–7462–0000–5 Series

Copyright

© 1988 by Kluwer Academic Publishers

All rights reserved. No part of this publication may be reproduced, stored in a retrieval system, or transmitted in any form or by any means, electronic, mechanical, photocopying, recording or otherwise, without prior permission from the publishers, Kluwer Academic Publishers BV, PO Box 17, 3300 AA Dordrecht, The Netherlands.

Published in the United Kingdom by Kluwer Academic Publishers,
PO Box 55, Lancaster, UK.

Kluwer Academic Publishers BV incorporates the publishing programmes of
D. Reidel, Martinus Nijhoff, Dr W. Junk and MTP Press.

Printed in Great Britain by
Butler & Tanner Ltd, Frome and London

CONTENTS

List of Authors	vi
Series Editor's Foreword	vii
About the Editor	viii
1. Hypercalcaemic Disorders *S. H. Ralston*	1
2. Hypercalciuria *V. L. Sharman*	33
3. Recurrent calculi *C. A. C. Charlton*	59
4. Cystinuria *R. S. C. Rodger*	73
Index	89

LIST OF AUTHORS

C. A. C. Charlton
Department of Urology
Royal United Hospital
Combe Park, Bath
BA1 3NG
UK

S. H. Ralston
University Department of Medicine
Glasgow Royal Infirmary
10 Alexandra Parade
Glasgow G31 2ER
UK

R. S. C. Rodger
Renal Units
Stobhill General Hospital and
Western Infirmary
Glasgow
UK

V. L. Sharman
Department of Renal Medicine
St. Mary's Hospital
Milton Road
Portsmouth, Hants PO3 6AD
UK

SERIES EDITORS' FOREWORD

Renal stone disease remains a common clinical problem. Patients may attend either medical or surgical clinics and not infrequently present as acute abdominal emergencies to general practitioners, physicians, surgeons and even gynaecologists. Recent urinary calculi continue to cause considerable morbidity despite the recent advances in our understanding of the pathogenesis of the different types of stones involved and despite improvements in treatment – by appropriate drug therapy, by ultrasound techniques and by lithotripsy.

This volume discusses the investigation and management of patients with calculus disease. Each chapter has been written by an experienced clinician and provides information of considerable relevance and importance for all doctors engaged in clinical practice. The technical developments of the last few years have clearly demonstrated that renal stone disease, even when recurrent, should be an uncommon cause of chronic renal failure. Knowledge of the recent developments in this field is important for all practising doctors and even more important for their patients.

G. R. D. CATTO

ABOUT THE EDITOR

Dr Graeme R. D. Catto is Reader in Medicine at the University of Aberdeen and Honorary Consultant Physician/Nephrologist to the Grampian Health Board. His current interest in transplant immunology was stimulated as a Harkness Fellow at Harvard Medical School and the Peter Bent Brigham Hospital, Boston, USA. He is a member of many medical societies including the Association of Physicians of Great Britain and Ireland, the Renal Association and the Transplantation Society. He has published widely on transplant and reproductive immunology, calcium metabolism and general nephrology.

1
HYPERCALCAEMIC DISORDERS

S. H. RALSTON

INTRODUCTION

Although most patients with calcium-containing renal stones are normocalcaemic, many hypercalcaemic disorders are associated with an increased risk of renal stone disease. These conditions are important to recognize, since their identification and treatment invariably corrects the tendency to renal stone formation. The initial section of this chapter deals with the presentation, investigation and treatment of hypercalcaemic states in general. Subsequently, specific hypercalcaemic disorders are discussed, with particular emphasis on those associated with renal stone disease (Table 1.1).

HYPERCALCAEMIA – PRESENTATION AND CLINICAL FEATURES

Hypercalcaemia has been recognized with increasing frequency in recent years, due to the widespread introduction of multichannel biochemical autoanalysers which routinely measure plasma calcium concentrations even when they have not been specifically requested by the clinician. Patients with mild hypercalcaemia ($<3.00\,\text{mmol}\,L^{-1}$) are usually asymptomatic, at least with respect to their raised plasma calcium level, and generally present with features of an unrelated medical condition. On the other hand, those with more severe hypercalcaemia often have symptoms which are directly attributable to the elevation in plasma calcium levels. In the kidney, moderate or severe hypercalcaemia ($>3.20\,\text{mmol}\,L^{-1}$) results in impairment of urinary

TABLE 1.1   Causes of hypercalcaemia

ENDOCRINE CONDITIONS
  Primary hyperparathyroidism*
  Thyrotoxicosis
  Addison's disease
  Phaeochromocytoma
  Acromegaly*

MALIGNANT DISEASE
  Any malignant tumour with or without bone metastases

GRANULOMATOUS CONDITIONS
  Sarcoidosis*
  Tuberculosis
  Coccidiomycosis
  Histoplasmosis
  Systemic candidiasis
  Eosinophilic granuloma
  Berryliosis

IATROGENIC OR DRUG RELATED
  Vitamin D intoxication*
  Milk-alkali syndrome*
  Lithium
  Vitamin A intoxication
  Parenteral nutrition

ASSOCIATED WITH RENAL FAILURE
  Recovery phase of acute renal failure
  Aluminium toxicity
  Tertiary hyperparathyroidism*

MISCELLANEOUS
  Familial benign hypercalcaemia
  Immobilization*

* Indicates an association with an increased risk of renal stone disease and/or nephrocalcinosis

concentrating ability, and increased urinary losses of electrolytes, such as sodium and potassium[1]. Clinically, these effects are manifest by polyuria, nocturia and polydipsia. In the gastrointestinal tract, hypercalcaemia may cause nausea, anorexia and vomiting, either directly or in association with acute pancreatitis. Constipation is also a common complaint, due to the depressant effect of hypercalcaemia on neuromuscular transmission. In the central nervous system, confusion, somnolence, depression and psychosis may occur, progressing to coma in patients with extreme hypercalcaemia. The combination of increased renal losses of water and electrolytes, reduced levels of fluid intake as the result of gastrointestinal symptoms and alteration in the conscious level may, in some cases, lead to the syndrome of hypercalcaemic crisis: a deteriorating spiral of hypercalcaemia, dehydration and impaired renal function, which, if untreated, culminates in acute renal failure and death.

There are few physical signs of hypercalcaemia, except on examination of the eyes, where a white band of corneal calcification may be seen as a streak at the 3 o'clock and 9 o'clock positions on the lateral and medial borders of the limbus. Band keratopathy, where there is a band of corneal calcification traversing the palpebral fissure is rare, as is conjunctival calcification where flecks of calcium become deposited in the conjunctival sac and set up an inflammatory reaction.

INVESTIGATION OF HYPERCALCAEMIA

Although this subject receives attention in the individual sections dealing with the disorders associated with hypercalcaemia, a few general points are considered here.

To confirm the presence of hypercalcaemia, more than one measurement of plasma ionized calcium or total calcium, adjusted for serum albumin concentration, should be made. This is, of course, unnecessary in patients with severe symptomatic hypercalcaemia, where immediate calcium-lowering treatment may be indicated. It is not essential routinely to measure levels of ionized calcium in hypercalcaemic patients, except in situations where the clinician has reason to believe that the albumin-adjusted levels may be inaccurate; examples would be in the presence of significant acid–base disturbance, in extreme hypoalbuminaemia or in plasma cell dyscrasias where the massive increase in serum globulins may occasionally bind significant quantities of calcium. Many reviewers have emphasized the importance of confirming the diagnosis of mild hypercalcaemia by repeated measurements of calcium on fasting blood samples. This is probably unnecessary, however, since the finding of hypercalcaemia after an oral calcium load may be indicative of an underlying abnormality, such as primary hyperparathyroidism (PHPT)[2].

The measurement of plasma immunoreactive PTH (iPTH) concentration is probably the single most important investigation currently available for the assessment of a hypercalcaemic patient. The finding of raised iPTH concentrations in a hypercalcaemic patient strongly suggests the diagnosis of PHPT, and, as such, generally obviates the need for extensive and laborious investigation for the many relatively rare non-parathyroid causes of hypercalcaemia. While the finding of undetectable iPTH levels suggests a non-parathyroid cause of hypercalcaemia, the interpretation of iPTH levels which fall *within* the normal range is more difficult. Even under hypercalcaemic conditions, there is an element of 'non-suppressible' PTH secretion, so that plasma iPTH levels may occasionally be detectable in patients with non-parathyroid hypercalcaemia[3]. Thus, while detectable iPTH levels in a hypercalcaemic patient may be construed as representing autonomous iPTH secretion by a parathyroid adenoma, low levels of iPTH may also be observed in patients with non-parathyroid hypercalcaemia[4] and in familial benign hypercalcaemia[5]. This emphasizes the importance of taking the clinical picture and other biochemical investigations into account when assessing patients with undiagnosed hypercalcaemia.

Other routine investigations may give valuable clues in the differential diagnosis of hypercalcaemia. A hyperchloraemic acidosis is strongly suggestive of PHPT, although it is important to emphasize that most patients with this diagnosis have no significant abnormality of acid–base status. While a metabolic alkalosis may be found in many non-parathyroid causes of hypercalcaemia, this finding should raise suspicion of the milk-alkali syndrome. Patients with very high alkaline phosphatase (AP) levels (>3 times the upper normal limit) usually turn out to have malignant hypercalcaemia with liver infiltration. In such cases, a concomitant elevation in serum-glutamyl transferase

(GGT) levels should indicate the hepatic origin of the enzyme. Elevations of AP in PHPT are usually mild or moderate (< 3 times normal) and are almost invariably accompanied by radiological evidence of osteitis fibrosa cystica on careful scrutiny of hand X-rays. The GGT level is, of course, normal in PHPT except in the presence of coincidental liver pathology. Occasionally, grossly elevated levels of bone-derived AP may be seen in hypercalcaemic patients; this is usually due to the coincidental occurrence of Paget's disease in patients with other causes of hypercalcaemia.

Measurements of urinary calcium excretion are of limited value except in patients with familial hypocalciuric hypercalcaemia (FHH), where the extreme hypocalciuria may provide the only differentiating feature from PHPT[5]. Calculation of renal tubular phosphate reabsorption (TmPO$_4$) is similarly of limited value: although TmPO$_4$ levels are reduced in PHPT, low levels are also seen with other causes of hypercalcaemia, such as malignancy and FHH. Nephrogenous cyclic AMP (NcAMP) measurements have also been used in the differential diagnosis of hypercalcaemia since levels are raised in patients with PHPT and suppressed in some other benign causes of hypercalcaemia[6]. Elevated levels of NcAMP may also be found in patients with malignant hypercalcaemia, however, thus limiting their value in differential diagnosis[4].

There are two hypercalcaemic disorders where radiology provides valuable diagnostic information. The first is in suspected PHPT, where the demonstration of subperiostial bone erosions on hand X-rays may provide rapid confirmation of the diagnosis (Figure 1.1). This technique is particularly valuable in patients with severe hypercalcaemia because of the delay involved in obtaining iPTH results. In most patients with PHPT, however, skeletal radiographs have a low diagnostic yield since less than 10% of patients with PHPT have radiologically-apparent bone disease. It is therefore logical to limit skeletal radiology to the investigation of hypercalcaemic patients in whom abnormalities are likely to be demonstrated: that is, those with high-normal or raised serum AP levels of bone origin.

A second group of patients who frequently show abnormalities on skeletal imaging are those with suspected malignancy. In this situation, the most useful screening test is a radionuclide bone scan since, with the exception of myeloma, this technique is much more sensitive than

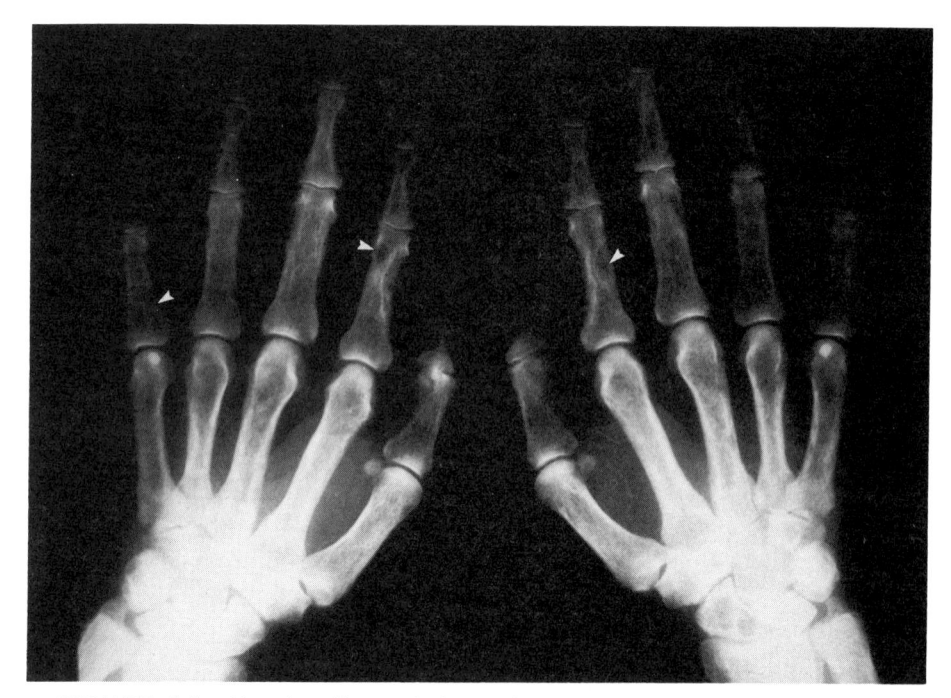

FIGURE 1.1 Hand radiograph in patient with severe PHPT showing florid subperiosteal erosions of bone in the phalanges and bone cysts (arrowed)

conventional radiology in detecting metastatic bone deposits[7].

MEDICAL MANAGEMENT OF HYPERCALCAEMIA

Since hypercalcaemia is not a disease in itself, the primary aims of management are to identify and treat the underlying disorder. In some cases, however, specific medical antihypercalcaemic therapy is indicated, either as a holding measure, to allow investigations to proceed, or to control the symptoms of hypercalcaemia when the underlying condition is untreatable.

Patients who merit urgent antihypercalcaemic therapy typically have serum calcium values of 3.50 mmol L^{-1} or greater, are dehydrated with impaired GRF and have prominent symptoms such as thirst, polyuria, nausea, vomiting, anorexia and confusion.

The first line of therapy in this situation is rehydration with intravenous fluids. A substantial reduction in plasma calcium values may be achieved in most cases by the intravenous infusion of 0.9% saline, 3–4 L daily for 24–48 h[8]. Thereafter, continued saline infusions of between 2–3 L daily should be administered to promote continued excretion of calcium in the urine. It is important to give sodium-containing intravenous fluids, rather than dextrose, in the rehydration of hypercalcaemic patients, since the excretion of calcium in the proximal renal tubule is directly related to that of sodium[1]. The calcium-lowering effect of a sodium diuresis has been further exploited in patients with severe hypercalcaemia by combining massive intravenous saline loads (>10 L daily) with high doses of loop diuretics[9]. This method of management is not recommended as a matter of routine, however, since it is associated with a significant risk of severe electrolyte imbalance and haemodynamic disturbance. It should only be used in conjunction with full intensive care facilities, including central venous pressure monitoring and regular measurement of urinary electrolyte losses. The use of loop diuretics in patients receiving more modest quantities of saline should be avoided, since this may actually reduce calcium excretion by causing sodium depletion.

In many cases, rehydration alone will be sufficient to stabilize the patient's condition; if not, specific antihypercalcaemic drug therapy is indicated. Most patients with severe hypercalcaemia which is unresponsive to rehydration have pathologically increased bone resorption. Intestinal calcium absorption seldom contributes significantly to the hypercalcaemia, if only because such patients are anorexic and taking little in the way of oral calcium in any case. Dietary calcium restriction is pointless in this situation; rather, drug therapy should be given with the aim of inhibiting bone resorptive activity.

The most rapidly acting agent currently available for the control of severe hypercalcaemia is intravenous infusion of neutral phosphate. Plasma calcium values start to fall within minutes of starting a phosphate infusion, due to acute precipitation of calcium–phosphate complexes in bone and soft tissues. There is, in addition, a more prolonged inhibitory effect on bone resorption[10]. Although highly effective, intravenous phosphate is limited in its application by serious adverse reactions, such as hypotension, acute renal failure and widespread metastatic calcification. Since these are particularly frequent in patients with hyperphosphataemia, phosphate therapy should be limited to those patients with severe hypercalcaemia and hypophosphataemia, in whom an immediate reduction in plasma calcium seems clinically imperative.

Calcitonin also has a rapid onset of action within 2–4 h of administration, due to inhibitory effects on osteoclastic bone resorption and renal tubular calcium reabsorption[11]. Although calcitonin is valuable in the acute situation, a proportion of patients fail to respond adequately, due to 'down regulation' of calcitonin receptors in the osteoclast after the first 48 h of treatment. Recent studies have shown, however, that the combination of calcitonin with other agents, such as corticosteroids or diphosphonates, may either prevent or circumvent this problem[12,13].

Mithramycin is an effective and reliable antihypercalcaemic drug. Given in the dose of 25 μg kg^{-1} body weight, it reduces plasma calcium values by inhibiting bone resorption and possibly by inhibiting renal tubular calcium reabsorption[14]. Although the onset of action is slower than calcitonin, plasma calcium values start to fall within 24 h and reach a nadir between 2–4 days. While hypercalcaemia can be controlled over a prolonged period by repeated mithramycin infusions, this carries the risk of serious adverse effects, such as thrombocytopaenia and drug-induced hepatitis. In the absence of pre-existing bone marrow suppression, however, up to three doses of mithramycin can usually be administered with safety.

The 'second generation' of diphosphonates, aminohydroxypropylidene diphosphonate (APD) and dichloromethylene diphosphonate (Cl$_2$MDP), although not yet generally available, are highly effective agents in the treatment of hypercalcaemia associated with increased bone resorption[15,16]. These drugs possess potent and sustained inhibitory effects on osteoclastic bone resorption, and, in recent studies, have been shown to be superior to mithramycin and the combination of calcitonin/corticosteroids[14]. While they have a relatively slow onset of action (24–48 h), combination with a rapidly acting agent, such as calcitonin, for the first few days of treatment may overcome this problem when a rapid hypocalcaemic effect is desired[12]. At present, the intravenous mode of administration is used because of poor absorption of diphosphonates in the gut. Indeed, this may explain the rather disappointing hypocalcaemic effect of oral ethane hydroxy diphosphonate (EHDP) – the only diphosphonate preparation currently available for routine clinical use. In most cases, the intravenous route does not cause too much inconvenience, however, since hypercalcaemia can in many cases be adequately controlled by intermittent diphosphonate infusions[17].

Although corticosteroids undoubtedly have a useful calcium lowering effect in some situations (sarcoidosis, vitamin D toxicity, lymphoreticular cancers), they cannot be recommended as a 'blanket' therapy for undiagnosed hypercalcaemia since they are generally ineffective in the two most common causes of hypercalcaemia: PHPT and hypercalcaemia associated with solid malignant tumours[18].

Oral phosphate[10] may be of value in some patients after the acute episode of hypercalcaemia has been controlled by parenteral agents. Although effective, its usefulness is limited by a high incidence of gastrointestinal effects. Like intravenous phosphate, it should not be given in the presence of hyperphosphataemia due to the risk of renal dysfunction and metastatic calcification.

PRIMARY HYPERPARATHYROIDISM

Introduction

Primary hyperparathyroidism (PHPT) is now recognized as a very common condition. Recent studies, based on biochemical screening of out-patients, indicate a prevalence of between 50–200 cases per 100 000 population[19,20]. Although uncommon in those under 40 years old, its incidence increases progressively thereafter, reaching a maximum in the seventh decade. Like most endocrine diseases, it is more common in women, particularly in the over-60 age group[19], where the female:male ratio approaches 7:1.

Pathogenesis

The syndrome of PHPT is due to the excessive and autonomous secretion of PTH by an enlarged mass of parathyroid tissue. In the vast majority of cases (80–90%), the cause is a benign enlargement of a single parathyroid gland[20]. Although multiple parathyroid adenomas do occur, this finding is usually seen when PHPT is part of a multiple endocrine neoplasia (MEN) syndrome. Carcinoma of the parathyroid is rare, accounting for less than 2% of patients with PHPT, but may be recognized clinically by its rapid onset, severe hypercalcaemia and florid bone changes.

A number of factors contribute to the pathogenesis of hypercalcaemia in PHPT; in the kidney, distal renal tubular reabsorption is increased, with the result that for any given level of serum calcium, urinary calcium excretion in PHPT is less than that in normal individuals with a similar degree of hypercalcaemia induced by calcium infusion (Figure 1.2)[21]. Although this elevation in renal tubular calcium reabsorption makes an important contribution to the pathogenesis of hypercalcaemia in PHPT, urinary calcium excretion is usually *elevated* in absolute terms due to the other metabolic effects of PTH: PTH stimulates increased renal production of $1,25(OH)_2D$, which, in turn, enhances intestinal calcium absorption[22]. In bone, PTH acts in conjunction with $1,25(OH)_2D$ to increase osteoclastic resorption. Although bone formation is also increased in PHPT, the net effect in most cases is in favour of resorption, leading to a negative skeletal calcium balance[23]. The combination of increased efflux of calcium from bone and increased intestinal calcium absorption results in chronic hypercalciuria with an increased risk of renal stone disease[22].

Presentation and clinical features

The mode of presentation in PHPT has changed dramatically over recent years, due to the advent of routine biochemical screening and increased recognition of patients with mild disease. Previous series of patients with PHPT contained a high proportion suffering from 'specific' complications, such as recurrent renal stone disease and osteitis fibrosa cystica. Nowadays, this mode of presentation is unusual: in a recent study[19], only 8% had renal stones, none had parathyroid bone disease and 57% were asymptomatic.

An important factor determining the occurrence of renal stone disease in PHPT is the patient's vitamin D status. In vitamin D replete subjects, the incidence of renal stone disease is high, due to the absorptive hypercalciuria associated with raised circulating levels of $1,25(OH)_2D$[22].

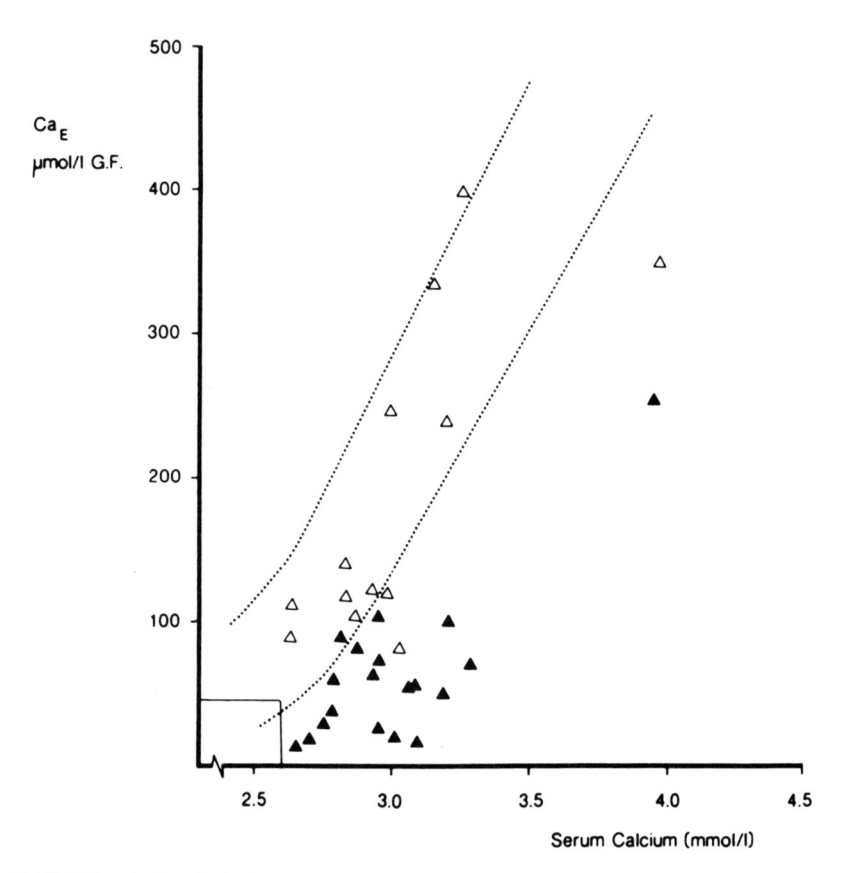

FIGURE 1.2 Relationship between serum calcium (adjusted for albumin) concentration and urinary calcium excretion expressed as a function of glomerular filtrate (Ca$_E$). The dotted lines indicate the 'normal' relationship, obtained by calcium infusion studies in control subjects[21]. In patients with PHPT (▲), urinary calcium excretion is lower than normals with an equivalent degree of hypercalcaemia, since PTH enhances renal tubular calcium reabsorption. Values in patients with 'bone resorptive' hypercalcaemia (△) due to immobilization, thyrotoxicosis and vitamin D intoxication generally fall within the normal range. *In absolute terms*, however, the urinary calcium excretion in PHPT is generally higher than that in normal fasting subjects (area enclosed by the solid lines in the bottom left hand corner)

When sensitive histomorphometric techniques are employed, minor increases in bone turnover are seen in many patients with PHPT[24]. Radiologically apparent bone disease is now rare, however, occurring in less than 10% of cases[20], again due to the increased recognition of patients with mild disease. Nowadays, by far the most common skeletal abnormality in patients with PHPT is osteoporosis. Since osteoporosis and PHPT are both common conditions in postmenopausal women, controversy surrounds the possible causal link between these conditions. Nonetheless, bone density is significantly reduced in PHPT when compared with age- and sex-matched controls[23], indicating that osteoporosis may be accelerated by PHPT, particularly in postmenopausal women, due to the more rapid rate of bone turnover[24].

The incidence of peptic ulceration in PHPT is high and it has been suggested that parathyroid overactivity may represent a risk factor for the development of peptic ulcer[25]. In some cases, there is a clear link between peptic ulceration and PHPT when Zollinger–Ellison syndrome may occur as part of an MEN 1 syndrome. In most cases, however, a causal relationship is unproven, since correction of hypercalcaemia seldom results in cure of the peptic ulcer disease.

Hypertension is a common feature of PHPT, with an incidence about twice that seen in age- and sex-matched controls[20]. The relationship between hypertension and PHPT is unclear, since the elevation in blood pressure does not invariably respond to surgical parathyroidectomy. This suggests an increased incidence of 'essential' hypertension in PHPT, rather than a specific effect of the increased serum calcium or PTH levels.

With the greatly increased recognition of PHPT, a variety of non-specific clinical features have appeared in association with the disease; these include fatigue, muscular weakness, vague musculoskeletal discomfort, depression and anxiety[26]. The relationship of such symptoms to the diagnosis of PHPT is unclear: they are usually present in patients with mild hypercalcaemia and respond variably to surgical parathyroidectomy, suggesting a chance association.

Investigation

The diagnosis of PHPT can, in most cases, be made on finding a raised or 'inappropriately detectable' level of iPTH in the presence of significant hypercalcaemia. Other abnormalities do occur, such as subperiosteal bone erosions, bone cysts, a 'pepperpot' skull on radiological screening and hyperchloraemic acidosis. These lend further weight to, but are by no means essential for the diagnosis. Indeed, the typical PHPT patient will nowadays present with no abnormalities other than hypercalcaemia, a low or low-normal phosphate level and a raised iPTH concentration. In all patients with suspected PHPT, it is advisable to measure the levels of urinary calcium excretion as low values may be the only clue to the diagnosis of familial hypocalciuric hypercalcaemia (FHH)[5].

In recent years, much interest has focussed on the preoperative localization of parathyroid adenomas in patients with suspected PHPT. Although it may be argued, with some justification, that neck exploration by an experienced parathyroid surgeon is the only localizing procedure necessary in PHPT, the development of newer, non-invasive imaging techniques has rekindled interest in this topic[27]. In some specialist centres, ultrasound scanning of the parathyroids has been found to be highly successful, although the general experience of this technique, and of CT scanning, has been disappointing. Perhaps the most promising of all the 'non-invasive' techniques currently available is the thyroid–parathyroid subtraction scan. This has the advantage of widespread availability, since it can be performed in any hospital with gamma camera facilities. Although accurate localization is obtained in about 70% of cases coming to surgery, this test should not be used in screening for the diagnosis of PHPT, since the scan may be negative in patients with mild PHPT. One further localization technique deserves mention: selective neck vein catheterization for iPTH measurements. Since this is an invasive and costly technique, there are only a few situations where it is indicated. One is in patients with a history of a previously failed neck exploration: surgery in such cases is technically difficult and the adenoma is often situated in the mediastinum. The value of preoperative localization, particularly in the latter situation, is self-evident. Other indications may include: patients with mild hypercalcaemia where peripheral venous iPTH measurements are equivocal; chronic renal failure with suspected tertiary hyperparathyroidism; and patients with another possible cause of hypercalcaemia, malignancy for example, in whom iPTH levels are detectable and the possibility of coexistent PHPT cannot be otherwise excluded.

Management

Surgical parathyroidectomy is the only effective treatment of PHPT. Until recently, most clinicians would have unhesitatingly advised parathyroidectomy in any patient with PHPT. However, the recognition of increasing numbers of asymptomatic patients with mild disease has called this practice into question. Many reports have appeared in the literature over recent years, showing that patients with mild PHPT, who were untreated for one reason or another, seldom developed problems related to the elevation in plasma calcium levels[28]. It is generally agreed that renal stone disease, parathyroid bone disease, severe symptomatic hypercalcaemia and significant renal impairment are absolute indications for parathyroidectomy. The role of surgery in patients who do not fit into one of these categories is more controversial, however, since there has been no study in which patients with asymptomatic PHPT have actually been randomized to receive surgical or conservative management. At present, many clinicians continue to advise parathyroidectomy in all patients, irrespective of symptoms, except when there are strong medical contraindications or in the very elderly. Since mild PHPT does not appear to be associated with any significant complications, however, another justifiable course of action is to adopt a conservative approach, especially if the patient does not welcome the prospect of a surgical operation and adequate follow-up can be arranged.

There is no effective medical treatment for PHPT at present: antihypercalcaemic therapy may, however, be employed to stabilize the condition of patients with severe hypercalcaemia prior to surgery. Long-term oral phosphate therapy has been used in some patients with PHPT: indications for this treatment are few since surgery should be advised in all symptomatic patients unless there are pressing contraindications. Oral phosphate should not be given to asymptomatic patients with PHPT because of the risk of side effects and the benign course of the untreated condition. Oestrogen therapy has been proposed as a means of preventing progression of osteoporosis in postmenopausal patients with PHPT[29]. Although oestrogens are certainly valuable in the prevention of postmenopausal osteoporosis (whether associated with PHPT or not), the hyperparathyroid state should still be treated surgically unless there are contraindications.

MALIGNANCY-ASSOCIATED HYPERCALCAEMIA

Incidence and epidemiology

This is by far the commonest cause of hypercalcaemia encountered in hospital practice and is second only to PHPT as a cause of hypercalcaemia in the general community. Hypercalcaemia is usually a feature of advanced malignant disease: in Fisken's series of 163 patients with cancer-associated hypercalcaemia, 75% had obvious metastases at the time of presentation[30]. Hypercalcaemia is not evenly distributed throughout the cancer population. Some common tumours, such as carcinoma of the stomach, large bowel and oat cell lung carcinoma, are rarely associated with hypercalcaemia (Table 1.2), whereas others, such as squamous bronchial carcinoma and breast carcinoma, are common causes. In tumours such as breast carcinoma and myeloma, the hypercalcaemia may be related to extensive metastatic bone involvement[31], but, in most solid tumours, there is no relationship between the extent of metastatic bone disease and plasma

TABLE 1.2 Tumour type in 190 patients presenting consecutively to Glasgow Royal Infirmary with malignant hypercalcaemia

Type of tumour	Percentage
Squamous bronchial carcinoma	35
Breast carcinoma	13
Myeloma/lymphoma	13.5
Genitourinary cancers	13.5
Oesophageal/head and neck (squamous)	10
Hepato-biliary cancer	3
Others	12

calcium values[32]. These differences almost certainly relate to the production and release of calcium-elevating humoral substances by some types of tumour tissue.

Pathogenesis

In some tumours, such as breast carcinoma or myeloma, hypercalcaemia may indeed arise as a consequence of extensive metastatic bone destruction, although this is usually combined with reduced urinary calcium excretion due to dehydration or renal failure. In the case of myeloma, increased bone resorption is mediated by the local release of lymphokines by the tumour cells, including interleukin-1, and tumour necrosis factors, alpha and beta, which have osteoclast-activating properties[31]. In breast carcinoma, locally active bone-resorbing factors are also released. Although the identity of these is less clear, possible candidates include the prostaglandins, epidermal growth factor and the tumour-derived growth factors[31].

In some lymphomas, hypercalcaemia and raised circulating levels of $1,25(OH)_2D$ are found, due to conversion of circulating $25(OH)D$ to the active metabolite in tumour tissue[33]. This contributes to the hypercalcaemia by raising intestinal calcium absorption and systemically stimulating bone resorption. Local release of osteoclast-activating lymphokines by tumour cells also contributes to the hypercalcaemia[31].

In solid tumours other than breast carcinoma, skeletal calcium release from bone metastases is seldom sufficient to cause hypercalcaemia[32]. Recent evidence suggests that, in these situations, the tumour releases a humoral factor, which is structurally distinct from PTH, yet mimics many aspects of PTH-like activity in bone and kidney[4,32,34]. Accordingly, these patients may have elevated urinary excretion of cAMP, low serum phosphate and $TmPO_4$ values, elevated renal tubular calcium reabsorption and, in some cases, raised $1,25(OH)_2D$ levels. The pathogenesis of hypercalcaemia is in many respects similar to that of PHPT. There are, however, two important differences: patients with malignant hypercalcaemia almost invariably have suppressed intestinal absorption of calcium, whether or not $1,25(OH)_2D$ levels are raised[34]. This may be due either to end organ resistance to the effects of $1,25(OH)_2D$ in malignancy or to production of a related metabolite with little or no metabolic activity. Secondly, as active bone formation is more depressed in the hypercalcaemia of malignancy than in PHPT, there is a much greater negative calcium balance for any given increase in bone resorption[35]. There is some suspicion that this 'uncoupling' of bone cell activity may be due to the effects of the transforming growth factors, rather than the PTH-like factors[36], although immobilization may also play a role in increasing bone resorption and depressing bone formation.

Presentation

Malignancy associated hypercalcaemia seldom presents a diagnostic problem, since most cancers are far advanced by the time hypercalcaemia becomes apparent. Accordingly, a thorough clinical history and examination will usually lead the clinician to the correct diagnosis. Although the humoral hypercalcaemia of malignancy shares certain biochemical features in common with PHPT, renal stone disease and radiological evidence of osteitis fibrosa cystica are almost never seen in malignancy, probably because the course of the disease is too rapid to permit the development of either complication.

Since squamous carcinoma of the bronchus is the commonest cause of malignancy associated hypercalcaemia, a chest X-ray is indicated as a routine in any patient with undiagnosed hypercalcaemia. Diagnostic abnormalities are invariably noted in patients with a bronchial primary, although further investigations may be necessary to determine the extent of tumour as surgical resection is occasionally possible. Patients with myeloma or other lymphoreticular cancers can usually be diagnosed by the combination of clinical features, immunoglobulin screening and bone marrow aspirate. Occasionally, in patients with suspected malignancy, the diagnosis is not obvious from clinical history or the above screening tests. In these patients, it is tempting to investigate the gastrointestinal tract first, since these patients usually have prominent gastrointestinal symptoms of hypercalcaemia. In fact, a primary gastric or colonic carcinoma seldom, if ever, presents in this way, and attention should be directed instead to more common 'occult' primary sites, such as the genitourinary tract, liver and nasopharynx (Table 1.2).

Management

There are two main objectives in the management of malignancy-associated hypercalcaemia. The first is to determine the tumour type and stage of progression in order to assess whether specific anticancer therapy may be helpful. The importance of this cannot be over-emphasized since effective treatment of the primary tumour is the only way of controlling malignant hypercalcaemia in the long term[14]. If anticancer treatment is not possible, medical treatment should be given to control symptoms related to the hypercalcaemia. Since accelerated bone resorption plays a major pathogenic role in most cases, drug therapy should be tailored accordingly[10-18]. Dietary calcium or vitamin D restriction is not likely to be of value, except in the case of some lymphomas where $1,25(OH)_2D$ levels are raised.

ENDOCRINE CAUSES OF HYPERCALCAEMIA

Thyrotoxicosis

Clinically important hypercalcaemia is rare in thyrotoxicosis, although mean concentrations of plasma calcium are higher in thyrotoxic patients than in normal individuals. In a recent study, only 4 out of 469 hospital patients with serum calcium values of $>2.80\,\text{mmol}\,L^{-1}$ were thyrotoxic[30].

The mechanisms of hypercalcaemia in thyrotoxicosis have recently been reviewed[37]: there is increased bone resorption, stimulated by the excessive amounts of circulating thyroid hormone. Although bone formation is also increased in thyrotoxic patients, resorption is elevated to a greater degree, leading to negative skeletal calcium balance and osteoporosis. The efflux of calcium from bone causes parathyroid gland suppression with depressed iPTH levels, depressed $1,25(OH)_2D$ levels, lowered intestinal absorption of calcium and raised serum phosphate and $TmPO_4$ values. Renal tubular reabsorption of calcium falls and this, in combination with increased bone resorption, causes hypercalciuria. Despite their elevated levels of urinary calcium excretion, patients with thyrotoxicosis seldom present with renal stone disease: the reasons for this are not clear but may be related to increased urinary excretion of inhibitors of stone formation or to the brief duration of the condition in its untreated state.

From the clinical point of view, thyrotoxicosis seldom presents a diagnostic problem: most patients are clearly thyrotoxic by the time hypercalcaemia has occurred. 'Masked thyrotoxicosis' may occasionally mimic malignancy-associated hypercalcaemia but thyroid function tests will usually reveal the correct diagnosis. Although thyrotoxic patients may occasionally present with severe hypercalcaemia and hypophosphataemia, either of these findings should raise the possibility of coexisting PHPT. In the majority of cases, treatment of the thyrotoxic state is all that is needed to correct the hypercalcaemia and other metabolic bone problems, although isolated patients may need specific antihypercalcaemic therapy while antithyroid treatment is taking effect.

Addison's disease

Hypercalcaemia is an occasional complication of untreated Addison's disease, occurring in about 6% of cases. The mechanisms of hypercalcaemia[38] are complex and include both (a) impairment of GFR and increased proximal renal tubular calcium reabsorption due to hypovolaemia and sodium depletion and (b) increased osteoclastic bone resorption related to the deficiency of glucocorticoids. Plasma iPTH and $1,25(OH)_2D$ levels are depressed and intestinal calcium absorption is reduced. Untreated patients may be hyperphosphataemic and hypocalciuric due to the impairment of GFR. The diagnosis is made on finding the typical clinical and biochemical features of Addison's disease in combination with hypercalcaemia. The hypercalcaemia is usually mild and can be rapidly reversed by saline infusion and hydrocortisone treatment.

Acromegaly

While hypercalcaemia is extremely rare in acromegaly, hypercalciuria is common, due to the combination of increased bone resorption and increased intestinal calcium absorption[39]. Because of the hypercalciuria and chronic course of the disease, the incidence of renal stone formation is increased. All of the calcium abnormalities return to normal with effective treatment of the endocrine problem. It should be emphasized that the occurrence of significant hypercalcaemia in an acromegalic patient should lead the clinician to suspect PHPT as part of the MEN 1 syndrome.

Phaeochromocytoma

The commonest cause of hypercalcaemia in phaeochromocytoma is PHPT as part of an MEN syndrome. However, it has been suggested that the increased hypercalcaemia may be caused, in some cases, by catecholamine secretion directly stimulating PTH secretion, and, in others, by a PTH-like substance produced by the tumour[40]. From the practical point of view, treatment of the adrenal lesion should take precedence. If hypercalcaemia remains after excision of the adrenal tumour, attention should be directed to the probable coexistence of PHPT.

GRANULOMATOUS DISEASES

Sarcoidosis

Abnormalities of calcium metabolism have long been recognized as a feature of sarcoidosis. Although patients with sarcoid were originally thought to have 'hypersensitivity' to vitamin D, it is now recognized that the hypercalcaemia and hypercalciuria is due to abnormal *metabolism* of 25(OH)D. Current evidence[41] suggests that the macrophages present in sarcoid granulomas can convert circulating 25(OH)D to the active metabolite, $1,25(OH)_2D$. Since the enzyme in sarcoid tissue escapes normal feedback control mechanisms, administration of even small amounts of vitamin D to patients with sarcoidosis results in unregulated and excessive production of $1,25(OH)_2D$[42].

The hypercalcaemia in sarcoidosis is mainly due to increased intestinal absorption of calcium as the result of the raised $1,25(OH)_2D$ levels. Bone resorption may also be elevated, however, due to the local release of calcium from skeletal sarcoidosis, or the systemic bone resorbing effects of $1,25(OH)_2D$. Typically, levels of iPTH are low and levels of plasma phosphate and $TmPO_4$, high. Hypercalciuria occurs as the result of increased intestinal absorption of calcium and reduced renal tubular calcium reabsorption due to suppression of PTH secretion[41].

Because of the chronic course of the disease and marked hypercalciuria, patients with sarcoidosis are at high risk of developing nephrolithiasis and nephrocalcinosis. Indeed, nephrocalcinosis is a much more common cause of renal failure in sarcoidosis than granulomatous involvement of the kidneys.

Sarcoidosis is one of the few causes of hypercalcaemia which responds adequately to corticosteroid therapy and, indeed, the presence of hypercalciuria or hypercalcaemia in sarcoidosis is a strong indication for steroid treatment. Steroids have two major effects in this situation. They correct the abnormal metabolism of vitamin D by suppressing the underlying granulomatous process[41]; in addition, they act directly on the intestine to inhibit calcium absorption[43]. Although most patients with sarcoid hypercalcaemia respond adequately to a short course of high-dose steroids (40–60 mg prednisolone daily), dietary calcium and vitamin D restriction are also advisable in patients with active disease. Recent studies have shown that antimalarial drugs, such as chloroquine, may also be effective in correcting the abnormalities of calcium homeostasis in sarcoidosis[41].

Tuberculosis

Although this is a rare cause of symptomatic hypercalcaemia in clinical practice, recent surveys have shown a 40% prevalence of mild hypercalcaemia in untreated tuberculosis[44]. The mechanisms of hypercalcaemia in this situation have not been studied extensively. However, as in the case of sarcoidosis, there is an exaggerated hypercalcaemic response to vitamin D administration. In the study cited above, all cases of hypercalcaemia were found to remit after withdrawal of low-dose vitamin D supplements. Although iPTH levels are low or undetectable in tuberculous hypercalcaemia, there are no reported measurements of $1,25(OH)_2D$ concentrations. It seems likely, however, that the hypercalcaemia in this situation is similar to that in sarcoidosis: increased conversion of circulating $25(OH)D$ to the active metabolite, $1,25(OH)_2D$, in tuberculous granulomas.

In most cases, tuberculous hypercalcaemia is mild and can be reversed simply by rehydration and withdrawal of vitamin D supplements. Persistent or severe hypercalcaemia should suggest another underlying pathology.

Other granulomatous conditions

Hypercalcaemia and hypercalciuria have been reported to occur in a number of other granulomatous diseases, including systemic candidiasis[45], histoplasmosis[46], coccidiomycosis[47], berylliosis[48] and eosinophilic granuloma[49]. Current evidence suggests that the pathogenesis is similar to that in sarcoidosis. In some of the conditions mentioned above, evidence of increased 'sensitivity' to vitamin D supplements, and/or raised circulating levels of $1,25(OH)_2D$ have been documented[45,46,49].

The hypercalcaemia can usually be controlled by treatment of the underlying disorder and rehydration. Corticosteroids may be of value in berylliosis and eosinophilic granuloma[46,47], but should be avoided in the other conditions because of their immunosuppressive effects.

IMMOBILIZATION

Prolonged immobilization is invariably associated with the development of hypercalciuria, osteoporosis and an increased risk of nephrolithiasis[50]. Hypercalcaemia, in contrast, is a relatively rare complication of immobility, due to homeostatic mechanisms which prevent hypercalcaemia at the expense of hypercalciuria. Immobilized patients rapidly enter a phase of negative skeletal calcium balance as an adaptive response to the decreased mechanical stresses on the skeleton. There is a generalized increase in osteoclastic bone resorption and decreased bone formation; iPTH and $1,25(OH)_2D$ secretion are suppressed, resulting in decreased intestinal calcium absorption, low rates of urinary cAMP excretion, elevated serum phosphate and $TmPO_4$ levels and reduced renal tubular calcium reabsorption. The combination of an increase in net bone resorption and the reduction in renal tubular calcium reabsorption results in marked hypercalciuria. Patients who become hypercalcaemic as the result of immobilization, however, usually have a pre-existing elevation in bone turnover: the further increase in bone resorption, uncoupled from bone formation releases a calcium load in excess of that which can be excreted by the kidney, causing plasma calcium values to rise. In adults, the only common situation where this arises is in patients with widespread Paget's disease, but adolescents or children who are immobilized develop hypercalcaemia more frequently, due to the higher rate of bone turnover in the growing skeleton. It is important to recognize that immobility may precipitate severe hypercalcaemia in patients with other disorders, such as PHPT, thyrotoxicosis and malignancy.

Since hypercalcaemia is rare in immobilization *per se*, it is best to investigate fully those patients who present with this problem: a significant number will turn out to have another underlying disorder of calcium metabolism.

With regard to management, it is seldom worth trying to prevent bone loss since the osteopaenia is fully reversible on returning to normal activity. In patients who remain paralysed, the rate of negative skeletal calcium balance diminishes with time and approaches zero by about 12 months, resulting in a degree of osteopaenia which is appropriate for the stresses experienced by the skeleton.

In most cases, a high fluid intake of at least 3 L daily should be advised during the early phase of immobilization to promote passage of a dilute urine and prevent urinary stone formation. In the event of severe or symptomatic hypercalcaemia, intravenous saline infusions should be given and an inhibitor of bone resorption administered to reduce temporarily the release of skeletal calcium.

DRUG-INDUCED HYPERCALCAEMIA

Vitamin D intoxication

This is the commonest cause of iatrogenic hypercalcaemia, typically occurring in patients with hypoparathyroidism, osteomalacia, chronic renal disease or osteoporosis, who are inadvertently given too large a dose of vitamin D or one of its analogues.

The hypercalcaemia of vitamin D intoxication is primarily due to a combination of increased intestinal calcium absorption and increased osteoclastic bone resorption. While vitamins D_2, D_3 and 25(OH)D have relatively weak calcium-elevating properties, they do possess significant effects when present in high concentrations. Although PTH secretion is suppressed in vitamin D toxicity, normal or raised 1,25(OH)$_2$D levels may be seen, due to a 'mass action' effect of the grossly elevated levels of the precursor on renal 1α-hydroxylation[51]. Patients with vitamin D toxicity commonly have a substantial impairment of GFR; much more so, for example, than patients with PHPT who have an equivalent degree of hypercalcaemia. There is some evidence to suggest that this profound deterioration in renal function may, in part, be due to a nephrotoxic effect of the vitamin D metabolites themselves[52], although the hyperphosphataemia associated with vitamin D intoxication also contributes to renal impairment by causing nephrocalcinosis. Rather surprisingly, symptomatic renal stone disease is unusual in vitamin D intoxication. This may be due to the fact that patients with significant toxicity tend to develop severe hypercalcaemia and renal failure rather than prolonged hypercalciuria.

The basic biochemical features of vitamin D intoxication are similar whatever metabolite is taken: the patient is hypercalcaemic, hyperphosphataemic and usually has substantial impairment of GFR. Plain radiographs may show nephrocalcinosis and extensive vascular calcification. Since the diagnosis is almost invariably made on the history, detailed investigations are usually unnecessary. An exception is in the case of surreptitious vitamin D ingestion where grossly elevated 25(OH)D levels are diagnostic[51].

The time taken for hypercalcaemia and hypercalciuria to reverse after therapy is withdrawn varies considerably, depending on which metabolite is taken[53]. With vitamin D itself and 25(OH)D, hypercalcaemia may persist for weeks or even months, whereas, with the more polar metabolites, 1α-(OH) vitamin D and 1,25(OH)$_2$D, reversal of hypercalciuria and hypercalcaemia is invariably seen within 2–14 days.

With the shorter acting sterols, withdrawal of therapy and rehydration is usually all that is needed. In vitamin D or 25(OH)D toxicity, however, additional treatment with corticosteroids (prednisolone, 40 mg daily, initially) may be necessary, along with dietary calcium restriction. In this situation, corticosteroids appear to act by reducing intestinal calcium absorption and inhibiting bone resorption[43,54].

Thiazide diuretics

Although thiazide administration has long been associated with hypercalcaemia, controversy continues to surround its very existence as a specific entity. It is currently considered that, in susceptible individuals, thiazides cause hypercalcaemia because proximal renal tubular calcium reabsorption is increased as the result of hypovolaemia and sodium depletion. However, it has been argued that the development of hypercalcaemia in a thiazide-treated patient almost invariably reflects the presence of an underlying disorder of calcium metabolism – usually PHPT[55]. The hypercalcaemia associated with thiazide administration is mild: plasma calcium values of more than 3.00 mmol/L^{-1} in thiazide-treated patients invariably reflect another underlying cause.

The typical patient is a middle-aged woman with thiazide-treated hypertension who is discovered to be hypercalcaemic on routine screening. The best course of action is to stop the drug for a period of 4–6 weeks and recheck plasma calcium. In many patients, the hypercalcaemia persists: most of these will turn out to have PHPT, and should be investigated accordingly. If hypercalcaemia reverses, it is traditional to withdraw thiazide medication, although the mild hypercalcaemia induced by thiazides would not be expected to cause significant morbidity in the long term.

Lithium

Chronic lithium administration has been reported to cause mild hypercalcaemia in about 10% of patients[56]. In a few cases, lithium causes an elevation of the 'set point' at which raised plasma calcium levels inhibit PTH secretion by the parathyroid gland, leading to a functional state of hyperparathyroidism. However, about 75% of patients with lithium-associated hypercalcaemia turn out to have true adenomatous PHPT. It is currently unclear whether these adenomas are actually the result of lithium treatment or a coincidental finding.

From the practical point of view, patients suspected of suffering from this condition should be investigated for PHPT, with particular emphasis on localization procedures. If the evidence points to a single adenoma, neck exploration should be advised. Since the consequences of stopping treatment are usually more severe than the effects of mild hypercalcaemia, lithium therapy can be continued in the remainder with regular monitoring of plasma calcium values.

Milk-alkali syndrome

This is now a rare cause of hypercalcaemia, probably because of the efficacy of H_2 antagonists in the treatment of peptic ulcer disease. It occurs when absorbable alkali is taken in combination with excessive quantities of calcium, usually in the form of 'over the counter' calcium-containing antacids[57]. The mechanisms of hypercalcaemia are twofold: there is increased absorption of calcium from the intestine and decreased urinary calcium excretion, due to the enhancement of renal tubular calcium reabsorption by the alkalosis. Nephrocalcinosis and renal failure are often prominent since the alkalosis enhances precipitation of insoluble calcium salts in soft tissue. Symptomatic renal stone disease is rare.

The diagnosis of milk-alkali syndrome is made by taking an accurate history, although if there is surreptitious antacid ingestion, the finding of a metabolic alkalosis may provide an important clue to the diagnosis. Treatment consists of rehydration and withdrawal of the antacid and calcium preparations.

Vitamin A toxicity

Hypercalcaemia is a rare complication of severe vitamin A intoxication, due to enhanced osteoclastic bone resorption stimulated by the retinoid[58]. Treatment is by rehydration and withdrawal of the vitamin. Inhibitors of bone resorption may also be of theoretical value if the patient fails to respond to the above measures.

Parenteral nutrition

Hypercalcaemia and hypercalciuria are well established complications of total parenteral nutrition[59]. The pathogenesis is at present unclear and the metabolic abnormalities persist even after vitamin D and calcium supplements are withdrawn. Levels of iPTH and $1,25(OH)_2D$ are low. In some cases, deposition of aluminium on mineralizing bone surfaces has been implicated, as has immobilization. Since the hypercalcaemia is usually mild, no specific treatment is indicated. In one patient who recently presented to our department with symptomatic hypercalcaemia, treatment with the diphosphonate, APD, was dramatically effective indicating that, in some cases, increased bone resorption may play an important pathogenic role.

FAMILIAL HYPOCALCIURIC HYPERCALCAEMIA

This is a rare, but important, condition since it is easily mistaken for PHPT on clinical and biochemical grounds[5]. Since it is inherited in an autosomal dominant fashion, affected individuals may have a family history of hypercalcaemia, or, more usually, failed neck explorations for presumed PHPT. In contrast to PHPT, patients with FHH never suffer side effects as the result of their hypercalcaemia.

Two definite abnormalities can be defined in these patients: there is increased renal tubular reabsorption of calcium with failure of the raised plasma calcium levels to suppress PTH secretion. FHH can therefore be considered as a condition in which there is a raised 'set point' for plasma calcium homeostasis.

Clinically, patients with FHH have mild to moderate hypercalcaemia in the absence of obvious symptoms. While levels of iPTH are often 'inappropriately' detectable, FHH can usually be distinguished[5] from PHPT by a ratio of urinary calcium to creatinine clearance below 0.01. The main reason for identification of FHH is to prevent the patient and the affected relatives from undergoing unnecessary parathyroid surgery: untreated patients suffer no ill effects as the result of their elevated plasma calcium concentrations.

HYPERCALCAEMIA ASSOCIATED WITH RENAL FAILURE

Hypercalcaemia is a frequent complication in patients with acute and chronic renal disease: in Fisken's series, these disorders accounted for 15% of all cases of hypercalcaemia in hospital patients[30]. The causes are diverse and include the recovery phase of acute renal failure, vitamin D intoxication, aluminium toxicity and tertiary hyperparathyroidism.

Hypercalcaemia in the recovery phase of acute renal failure is usually seen in patients with crush injuries and myoglobinuria. It is thought that large amounts of calcium are taken up by damaged muscle tissue in the oliguric phase and that this is released during the diuretic phase[60]. Since the hypercalcaemia is mild and self limiting, no therapy is necessary.

Hypercalcaemia has recently been described in patients receiving haemodialysis, due to excessive accumulation of aluminium at the calcificiaton front in mineralizing osteoid. While these patients may be thought to have tertiary hyperparathyroidism, aluminium toxicity can be distinguished by lower levels of iPTH and AP, high plasma aluminium concentrations and demonstration of aluminium deposits in mineralizing bone[61]. The hypercalcaemia can be treated by stopping oral aluminium-containing phosphate binders, reducing the aluminium content of the dialysis water and dialysing against a low calcium concentration in the dialysate. Concurrent vitamin D therapy should, of course, also be stopped.

In chronic renal failure, plasma calcium values tend to fall as the result of hyperphosphataemia and reduced intestinal calcium reabsorption due to failure of $1,25(OH)_2D$ production[62]. The normal adaptive response to this situation is parathyroid gland hypertrophy, with increased secretion of iPTH, which tends to restore normocalcaemia by mobilizing calcium from bone and increasing phosphate excretion. On occasion, this process of secondary hyperparathyroidism overcompensates, resulting in the syndrome of tertiary hyperparathyroidism (THPT). The diagnosis in these patients is usually easy: typically, the patient has a long history of chronic renal failure and is usually on maintenance haemodialysis. Plasma iPTH levels are grossly elevated; the patient is hypercalcaemic, hyperphosphataemic and often has substantially raised AP levels. Skeletal radiographs usually reveal florid parathyroid bone disease. Localization procedures show enlargement of all four parathyroid glands and patients should be treated by subtotal parathyroidectomy. Hypercalcaemia and raised iPTH levels in patients with mild or moderate chronic renal failure are almost invariably due to PHPT rather than THPT. These patients should, of course, be treated by excision of the single adenoma.

A special situation where THPT becomes apparent is after renal transplantation, when hypercalcaemia is often precipitated by the sudden restoration of normal phosphate and vitamin D metabolism by the functioning kidney. While the parathyroid glands are slow to respond to the hypercalcaemia, they usually involute over a period of weeks or months after renal transplant. Parathyroidectomy is not routinely indicated, but may be necessary if the condition fails to correct itself spontaneously.

References

1. Benabe, J. E. and Martinez-Maldonado, M. (1978). Hypercalcaemic nephropathy. *Arch. Intern. Med.*, **38**, 777–9
2. Broadus, A. E., Horst, R. L., Littledike E. T., Mahaffey, J. E. and Rasmussen, H. (1980). Primary hyperparathyroidism with intermittent hypercalcaemia: serial observations and simple diagnosis by means of an oral calcium tolerance test. *Clin. Endocrinol.*, **12**, 225–35
3. Miajer, G. P., Keaton, J. A., Hurst, J. G. and Habener, J. F. (1979). Effect of plasma calcium concentration on relative proportion of intact hormone and carboxyl fragments in parathyroid venous blood. *Endocrinology*, **104**, 1778–84
4. Stewart, A. F., Horst, R., Deftos, L. J., Cadman, E. C., Lang, R. and Broadus, A. E. (1980). Biochemical evaluation of patients with cancer-associated hypercalcaemia – evidence for humoral and non-humoral groups. *N. Engl. J. Med.*, **303**, 1377–83.
5. Menko, F. H., Bijvoet, O. L. M., Fronen, J. L. H. H., Sandler, L. M., Adami, S., O'Riordan, J. L. H. and Schopman, W. (1983). Familial benign hypercalcaemia – study of a large family. *Q. J. Med.*, **206**, 120–40
6. Broadus, A. E., Mahaffey, J. E., Barrter, F. C. and Neer, R. M. (1977). Nephrogenous cyclic adenosine monophosphate as a parathyroid function test. *J. Clin. Invest.*, **60**, 771–83
7. Roberts, J. G., Gravelle, I. H., Baum, M., Bligh, A. S., Leach, K. G. and Hughes, L. E. (1976). Evaluation of radiography and skeletal scintigraphy for detecting skeletal metastases in breast carcinoma. *Lancet*, **1**, 273–6
8. Hosking, D. J., Cowley, A. and Bucknall, C. A. (1981). Rehydration in the treatment of severe hypercalcaemia. *Q. J. Med.*, **50**, 473–81
9. Suki, W. N., Yuimm, J. J., von Minden, M. *et al.* (1970). Acute treatment of

hypercalcaemia with furosemide. *N. Engl. J. Med.*, **283**, 836–40
10. Goldsmith, R. S. and Ingbar, S. H. (1966). Inorganic phosphate treatment of hypercalcaemia of diverse aetiologies. *N. Engl. J. Med.*, **274**, 1–7
11. Hosking, D. J. and Gilson, D. (1984). Comparison of the renal and skeletal actions of calcitonin in the treatment of severe hypercalcaemia of malignancy. *Q. J. Med.*, **211**, 359–69.
12. Ralston, S. H., Alzaid, A. A., Gardner, M. D. and Boyle, I. T. (1986). Treatment of cancer-associated hypercalcaemia with combined aminohydroxypropylidene diphosphonate and calcitonin. *Br. Med. J.*, **292**, 1549–50
13. Binstock, M. L. and Mundy, G. R. (1980). Effect of glucocorticoids and calcitonin in combination in malignant hypercalcaemia. *Ann. Intern. Med.*, **93**, 269–72
14. Ralston, S. H., Gardner, M. D., Dryburgh, F. J., Jenkins, A. S., Cowan, R. A. and Boyle, I. T. (1985). Comparison of aminohydroxypropylidene diphosphonate, mithramycin and corticosteroids/calcitonin in treatment of cancer-associated hypercalcaemia. *Lancet*, **2**, 907–10
15. Sleeboom, H. P., Bijvoet, O. L. M., Van Oosteroom, A. T., Gleed, J. H. and O'Riordan J. L. H. (1983). Comparison of intravenous (3-amino-1-hydroxypropylidene)-1, 1-bisphosphonate and volume repletion in tumour-induced hypercalcaemia. *Lancet*, **1**, 239–43
16. Jung, A. (1982). Comparison of two parenteral diphosphonates in hypercalcaemia of malignancy. *Am. J. Med.*, **72**, 221–6
17. Cantwell, B. M. J. and Harris, A. L. (1987). Effect of single high dose infusions of aminohydroxypropylidene diphosphonate on hypercalcaemia caused by cancer. *Br. Med. J.*, **294**, 467–70
18. Percival R. C., Yates, A. J. P., Gray, R. E. S., Forrest, A. W. and Kanis, J. (1984). Role of glucocorticoids in the management of malignant hypercalcaemia. *Br. Med. J.*, **289**, 287
19. Mundy, G. R., Cove, D. H. and Fisken, R. (1980). Primary hyperparathyroidism: changes in the pattern of clinical presentation. *Lancet*, **1**, 1317–20
20. Heath, H., Hodgson, S. F. and Kennedy, M. A. (1980). Primary hyperparathyroidism: incidence, morbidity and potential economic impact on a community. *N. Engl. J. Med.*, **302**, 189–93
21. Peacock, M., Robertson, W. G. and Nordin, B. E. C. Relation between serum and urinary calcium with particular reference to parathyroid activity. *Lancet*, **1**, 384–8
22. Broadus, A. E., Horst, R. L., Lang, R., Littledike, E. T. and Rasmussen, H. (1980). The importance of circulating 1,25 dihydroxyvitamin D and renal stone formation in primary hyperparathyroidism. *N. Engl. J. Med.*, **302**, 421–6
23. Pak, C. Y. C., Stewart, A., Kaplan, R., Bone, H., Notz, C. and Browne, R. (1975). Photon absorptiometric analysis of bone density in primary hyperparathyroidism. *Lancet*, **2**, 7–8
24. Meunier, P., Vignon, G., Bernard, J. *et al.* (1973). Quantitative bone histology as applied to the diagnosis of hyperparathyroid states. In Frame, B., Parfitt, A. M. and Duncan, H. (eds.) *Clinical Aspects of Metabolic Bone Disease*, pp. 215–25. (Amsterdam: Excerpta Medica)
25. Barreras, R. F. (1973). Calcium and gastric acid secretion. *Gastroenterology*, **64**, 1168–84
26. Aurbach, G. D., Mallette, L. E., Patten, B. M., Heath, D. A., Dippman, J. L. and Bilzikian, J. P. (1973). Hyperparathyroidism; recent studies. *Ann. Intern. Med.*, **79**, 556–81

27. McKillop, J. H., Boyle, I. T., Gunn, I. G., and Hutchison, J. S. F. (1986). Preoperative localisation of parathyroid adenomas. *Scott. Med. J.*, **31**, 10–15
28. Scholz, D. A., and Purnell, D. C. (1981). Asymptomatic primary hyperparathyroidism: 10 year prospective study. *Mayo Clin. Proc.*, **56**, 473–8
29. Selby, P. L. and Peacock, M. (1986). Ethinyl estradiol in the treatment of primary hyperparathyroidism in postmenopausal women. *N. Engl. J. Med.*, **314**, 1481–5
30. Fisken, R., Heath, D. A. and Bold, A. M. (1980). Hypercalcaemia – a hospital survey, *Q. J. Med.*, **196**, 405–18
31. Mundy, G. R. (1985). Pathogenesis of hypercalcaemia of malignancy. *Clin. Endocrinol. (Oxf.)*, **23**, 705–14
32. Ralston, S. H., Fogelman, I., Gardner, M. D. and Boyle, I. T. (1984). Relative contribution of humoral and metastatic factors to the pathogenesis of hypercalcaemia in malignancy. *Br. Med. J.*, **288**, 1405–8
33. Davies, M., Hayes, M. E., Mawer, E. B. and Lumb, G. A. (1985). Abnormal vitamin D metabolism in Hodgkin's lymphoma. *Lancet*, **2**, 1186–8
34. Ralston, S. H., Cowan, R. A., Gardner, M. D., Fraser, W. D., Marshall, E. and Boyle, I. T. (1987). Comparison of intestinal calcium absorption and circulating 1,25 dihydroxyvitamin D levels in malignancy associated hypercalcaemia and primary hyperparathyroidism. *Clin. Endocrinol. (Oxf.)*, **26**, 281–91
35. Stewart, A. F., Vignery, A. M., Silvergate, A. *et al.* (1982). Quantitative bone histomorphometry in humoral hypercalcaemia of malignancy; uncoupling of bone cell activity. *J. Clin. Endocrinol. Metab.*, **55**, 219–27
36. D'Souza, S. M., Ibbotson, K. J. and Mundy, G. R. (1984). Failure of parathyroid hormone antagonists to inhibit the in vitro bone resorptive activity produced by two animal models of humoral hypercalcaemia of malignancy. *J. Clin. Invest.*, **74**, 1104–7
37. Auwerx, J. and Boullion, R. (1986). Mineral and bone metabolism in thyroid disease: a review. *Q. J. Med.*, **232**, 737–52
38. Muls, E., Boullion, R., Boelart, J. *et al.* (1982). Etiology of hypercalcaemia in Addison's disease. *Calcif. Tiss. Int.*, **34**, 523–6
39. Lund, B., Eskildsen, P. C., Lund, B. *et al.* (1981). Calcium and vitamin D metabolism in acromegaly. *Acta Endocrinol.* **96**, 444–50
40. Stewart, A. F., Hoecker, J. L., Mallette, L. E., Segre, G. V., Armatruda, T. T. and Vignery, A. (1985). Hypercalcaemia in phaeochromocytoma. *Ann. Intern. Med.*, **102**, 776–9
41. Singer, F. R. and Adams, J. S. (1986). Abnormal calcium homeostasis in sarcoidosis. *N. Engl. J. Med.*, **315**, 755–7
42. Papapoulos, S. E., Clemens, T. L., Fraher, L. J. *et al.* (1979). 1,25 Dihydroxycholecalciferol in the pathogenesis of the hypercalcaemia of sarcoidosis. *Lancet*, **1**, 627–30
43. Kimberg, D. B., Baerg, R. D. and Gershon, E. (1971). Effect of cortisone treatment on the active transport of calcium by the small intestine. *J. Clin. Invest.*, **50**, 1309–21
44. Abbasi, A. A., Chemplavil, J. K., Farah, S., Muller, B. F. and Ainstein, A R. (1979). Hypercalcaemia in active pulmonary tuberculosis. *Ann. Intern. Med.*, **90**, 324–8
45. Kantarjian, H. M., Saad, M. F., Estey, E. H., Sellin, R. V. and Samaan, N. A. (1983). Hypercalcaemia in systemic candidiasis. *Am. J. Med.*, **74**, 721–4

46. Murray, J. J. and Heim, C. R. (1985). Hypercalcaemia in disseminated histoplasmosis; aggravation by vitamin D. *Am. J. Med.*, **78**, 881–4
47. Parker, M. S., Dokoh, S., Woolfenden, J. M. and Buchsbaum, H. W. (1984). Hypercalcaemia in coccidiomycosis. *Am. J. Med.*, **76**, 341–4
48. Stoeckle, J. D., Hardy, G. L. and Weber, A. L. (1969). Chronic beryllium disease: long term follow up of sixty cases and selective review of the literature. *Am. J. Med.*, **46**, 545–61
49. Jurney, T. H. (1984). Hypercalcaemia in a patient with eosinophilic granuloma. *Am. J. Med.*, **76**, 527–8
50. Stewart, A. F., Adler, M., Byers, C. M., Segre, G. V. and Broadus, A. E. (1982). Calcium homeostasis in immobilisation: an example of resorptive hypercalciuria. *N. Engl. J. Med.*, **306**, 1136–40
51. Mawer, E. B., Hann, J. T., Berry, J. L. and Davies, M. (1985). Vitamin D. metabolism in patients intoxicated with ergocalciferol. *Clin. Sci.*, **68**, 135–41
52. Christiansen, C., Rodbro, P., Christensen M. S. *et al.* (1978). Deterioration of renal function during treatment of chronic renal failure with 1,25 dihydroxycholecalciferol. *Lancet*, **2**, 700–3
53. Kanis, J. and Russell, R. G. G. (1977). Rate of reversal of hypercalcaemia and hypercalciuria induced by vitamin D and its one alpha hydroxylated derivatives. *Br. Med. J.*, **1**, 78–81
54. Streck, W. F., Waterhouse, C. and Haddad, J. (1979). Glucocorticoid effects in vitamin D intoxication. *Arch. Intern. Med.*, **139**, 974–7
55. Christensson, T., Hellstrom, K. and Wengle, B. (1977). Hypercalcaemia and primary hyperparathyroidism. *Arch. Intern. Med.*, **137**, 1138–42
56. Ananth, J. and Dubin, S. E. (1983). Lithium and symptomatic hyperparathyroidism. *J. Soc. Med.*, **76**, 1026–9
57. Orwoll, E. S. (1982). The milk-alkali syndrome – current concepts. *Ann. Intern. Med.*, **97**, 242–9
58. Wieland, R. G., Hendricks, F. H., Leon, F. A. Y., Gutierrez, L. and Jones, J. C. (1971). Hypervitaminosis A with hypercalcaemia. *Lancet*, **1**, 698
59. Shike, M., Harrison, J. E., Sturtridge, W. C. *et al.* (1980). Metabolic bone disease in patients receiving long term total parenteral nutrition. *Ann. Intern. Med.*, **92**, 343–50
60. Llach, F., Felsenfeld, A. J. and Haussler, M. R. (1981). The pathophysiology of altered calcium metabolism in rhabdomyolysis-induced acute renal failure. *N. Engl. J. Med.*, **305**, 117–23
61. Boyce, B. F., Fell, G. S., Elder, H. Y. *et al.* (1982). Hypercalcaemic osteomalacia due to aluminium toxicity. *Lancet*, **2**, 1009–13
62. Kanis, J. A. (1985). Renal bone disease. In Weatherall, D. J., Ledingham, J. G. G. and Warrell, D. A. (eds.) *Oxford Textbook of Medicine*, Vol. 2, pp. 18.136–43. (Oxford: Oxford University Press)

2
HYPERCALCIURIA

V. L. SHARMAN

The majority of patients who form stones within the urinary tract have an associated metabolic disorder. A relationship between the increased excretion of calcium in the urine in patients with renal and ureteric calculi was first noted by Flocks[1,2] but it was Albright[3] who, in 1953, first coined the term 'idiopathic hypercalciuria', suggesting that the condition might have a tubular origin and drawing attention to the hypophosphataemia which is often present. A few years later, Henneman *et al.*[4] demonstrated high calcium absorption, and, subsequently, Jackson and Dancaster[5] suggested that this hyperabsorption was an adaptation to the increased urinary calcium loss. No cause can be identified in nearly all normocalcaemic hypercalciuric patients and an autosomal dominant mode of inheritance has been suggested[6]. The prevalence of hypercalciuria is approximately 5% in otherwise normal adults, and, in 95% of these subjects, hypercalciuria is silent and not associated with stone formation.

NORMAL PHYSIOLOGY

Daily dietary calcium intake varies from 5–50 mmol with an average of 20 mmol. Active transport is the major mechanism of intestinal calcium absorption with only 15% of calcium being absorbed by simple diffusion. In a normal adult in calcium balance, bone resorption and bone mineralization result in the release and utilization of equivalent amounts of calcium, and, therefore, do not influence net calcium entry into the extracellular pool. The renal tubule plays the dominant role in short-term calcium homeostasis, minute-to-minute calcium excretion being dependent on the relationship between the rate of glomerular filtration and tubular reabsorption. Longer-term calcium excretion reflects the rates of intestinal absorption or bone resorption, processes which are controlled by parathyroid hormone and 1,25 dihydroxycholecalciferol ($1,25(OH)_2D_3$). The filtered load of calcium is approximately 200 mmol per day; 98% of this is reabsorbed leaving an average daily urinary calcium excretion of 4 mmol.

Direct sampling of glomerular filtrate in Bowman's capsule demonstrates a calcium concentration of 60% of that found in serum. Thus, slightly more than half the calcium in serum is not bound to plasma proteins and is filtered at the glomerulus. Reabsorption of calcium occurs along the proximal convoluted tubule in approximate proportion to that of sodium and water, the proximal tubular epithelium being highly permeable to calcium. The thin limb of Henle's loop is relatively impermeable to calcium but the thick ascending limb is a major site of calcium reabsorption. Evidence about the role of parathyroid hormone in this process is conflicting. 90% of calcium reabsorption occurs proximally, the predominant feature being its close relationship to sodium reabsorption. Factors which enhance sodium reabsorption in the proximal tubule enhance and factors which diminish tubular sodium reabsorption reduce proximal calcium reabsorption[7].

In the segments of the nephron beyond the loop of Henle, active calcium transport occurs but it is almost entirely dissociated from sodium reabsorption. In the distal convoluted tubule, which is relatively impermeable to calcium, calcium reabsorption is stimulated by parathyroid hormone[8] which also increases calcium absorption in the granular portion of the cortical collecting tubule[9].

EFFECT OF DIET ON CALCIUM EXCRETION

Calcium

Daily urinary excretion rises from an average of 2 mmol, when dietary calcium intake is less than 5 mmol, to 12 mmol, when intake increases to 150 mmol with calcium supplements. When intake is normal (5–50 mmol), excretion varies widely but seldom exceeds 7 mmol in normal subjects. If dietary calcium intake is varied, even by amounts as large as 50 mmol per day, urinary calcium excretion alters only by an average of 6%. Thus, changes in dietary calcium cause only very small changes in urinary calcium excretion in normal individuals. In contrast, the majority of patients with hypercalciuria display a marked increase in calcium excretion on a high-normal calcium intake[10].

The effect of a change in dietary calcium in altering urinary calcium is determined by the degree of intestinal calcium absorption, a process which has two components. Active transport of calcium is controlled by $1,25(OH)_2D_3$, and passive diffusion of calcium also occurs across a concentration gradient which is vitamin D independent. When dietary intake of calcium is normal, calcium absorption correlates closely with the plasma concentration of $1,25(OH)_2D_3$. In anephric patients who lack the enzyme to form $1,25(OH)_2D_3$, net intestinal absorption of calcium does not occur at normal levels of dietary calcium. However, absorption of calcium can be detected in such patients when dietary calcium is increased to 100 mmol per day.

Changes in dietary calcium alter urinary calcium excretion by changing both the filtered load of calcium and the secretion of parathyroid hormone. Since calcium deprivation lowers the serum calcium concentration and loading with calcium raises it, the consequent fall or rise in the filtered load of calcium may account, in part, for the subsequent fall or rise in urinary calcium. However, changes in renal tubular reabsorption of calcium resulting from altered parathyroid hormone secretion may be more important. Therefore, when dietary calcium increases and serum calcium rises, parathyroid hormone is suppressed, resulting in reduced calcium reabsorption and increased excretion. In contrast, when intake of calcium falls and serum calcium declines, urinary calcium excretion is reduced by a fall in filtered calcium and an increase in serum parathyroid hormone. These changes in parathyroid hormone occur within 24 h of a change in dietary calcium. In addition, increased calcium intake is accompanied by a fall in plasma $1,25(OH)_2D_3$, and reduced intake by a rise in plasma $1,25(OH)_2D_3$, these changes occurring within 36 h of the change in intake. Changes in plasma $1,25(OH)_2D_3$ are directly related to the preceding changes in serum parathyroid hormone and are reciprocally related to changes in the ratio of urinary calcium excretion to creatinine: plasma $1,25(OH)_2D_3$ falls as urinary calcium rises, and rises as urinary calcium falls. Thus, dietary calcium, by influencing parathyroid and vitamin D endocrine systems, helps to determine the capacity of the intestinal transport system to absorb a subsequent meal that contains calcium.

Protein

Stone disease is more prevalent in developed countries and increases in affluent societies. The composition of the diet is closely related to the level of affluence in a given population, the correlation being closest for consumption of animal protein. Thus, the incidence of stones in a given population might be related to the amount of animal protein in its diet. This hypothesis is supported by the observations that stone formers do ingest more animal protein, particularly that derived from meat, fish and poultry, and that the prevalence of stones among vegetarians is less than half that in the general population[11]. An increase in protein intake from $0.5\,\text{g}\,\text{kg}^{-1}\,\text{day}^{-1}$ to $2\,\text{g}\,\text{kg}^{-1}\,\text{day}^{-1}$ doubles calcium excretion in normal individuals[12]. Sulphur-containing amino acids raise urinary calcium[13], and the content of these amino acids in animal proteins is markedly higher than that in protein derived from vegetable origin. Eggs ($5.2\,\text{g}\,(100\,\text{g}\,\text{protein})^{-1}$), meat ($3.7\,\text{g}\,(100\,\text{g}\,\text{protein})^{-1}$) and particularly fish ($14.1\,\text{g}\,(100\,\text{g}\,\text{protein})^{-1}$) have a considerably higher content of sulphur-containing amino acids than do potatoes (2.9%), peas (2%) and beans (2.6%). These findings may explain why urinary calcium excretion is more closely related to animal protein than to overall protein consumption. High dietary protein results in increased urinary excretion associated with negative calcium balance[14] suggesting that the calcium is derived from bone. This effect may result from the increased acid production and excretion that accompanies high protein intake.

Phosphate

When daily dietary phosphate is greater than 10 mmol, urinary calcium is variable but does not exceed 7 mmol per day. However, severe phosphate depletion causes a reduction in tubular calcium reabsorption and hypercalciuria[15]. The increased urinary calcium is derived partly from increased intestinal absorption by increased $1,25(OH)_2D_3$ levels[16]. Skeletal resorption also contributes to the hypercalciuria as, in more prolonged dietary phosphate deprivation in animals, bone loss occurs. Animal studies show that neither parathyroidectomy nor vitamin D deficiency prevents the calciuric response to dietary phosphate deprivation, and, therefore, the augmented calcium excretion is independent of these endocrine systems. It is uncertain whether the milder degree of hypophosphataemia that occurs in primary hyperparathyroidism, idiopathic hypercalciuria or distal tubular acidosis contributes to the hypercalciuria in these disorders.

Other dietary factors

There is some evidence that urinary calcium increases by 0.6 mmol per 100 mmol increment in urinary sodium excretion. The clinical significance of this relatively small change in calcium excretion is unclear.

Urinary calcium rises acutely after administration of glucose, the result of reduced net tubular reabsorption of calcium[17]. This effect, which is insulin independent, is exaggerated in patients with idiopathic hypercalciuria. The clinical significance of this finding is also unclear.

METABOLIC ACIDOSIS AND ALKALOSIS

Metabolic acidosis is associated with the inhibition of tubular calcium reabsorption, thereby causing hypercalciuria[18]. This effect is largely independent of parathyroid hormone but it has been shown that acidosis may inhibit the effect of parathyroid hormone on calcium reabsorption[19]. Conversely, metabolic alkalosis is associated with enhanced calcium reabsorption and recent evidence has suggested that increased luminal bicarbonate concentration may enhance calcium reabsorption independently of systemic alkalosis[20]. This effect may, in part, account for the reduced incidence of hypercalciuria and renal calculi in proximal (type 2) renal tubular acidosis, compared with distal (type 1) renal tubular acidosis. In distal renal tubular acidosis, the unopposed effect of systemic metabolic acidosis is to decrease tubular calcium reabsorption which contributes to the hypercalciuria. It has been shown that the increased urinary calcium excretion following ammonium chloride-induced acidosis is the result of bone resorption.

SEASONAL VARIATIONS

Several studies have shown a marked seasonal variation in calcium excretion which reaches a maximum in July and August and a minimum in December and January[21]. As it has also been shown that irradiation of the skin will raise calcium excretion, it is possible that the seasonal effect is the result of sunlight stimulating $1,25(OH)_2D_3$ production during the summer months.

DEFINITION OF HYPERCALCIURIA

The term hypercalciuria implies that the 24 h urinary calcium on a free diet is higher than normal. However, the normal range of urinary calcium varies greatly in different parts of the world and hypercalciuria, as defined in certain countries or races, might be perfectly normal in others. Any particular definition of normality is therefore only applicable to a particular population group. Even such a definition may not be totally sound because there is evidence that calcium excretion has risen during the past 20 years and may even differ in different parts of the United Kingdom at any one time. Moreover, calcium excretion is not normally distributed but positively skewed making statistical analysis of data difficult. This has been examined by Robertson and Morgan[22] who found that the asymmetry in males is due to a distortion at the lower end of the distribution, there being a lower limit below which urinary calcium does not fall. The distribution of values above the mean is normal but below the mean is distorted.

Another factor complicating the recognition of hypercalciuria is the great intra-individual variation in urinary calcium. In patients on a free diet, urinary calcium may vary considerably from day to day or week to week, moving in and out of the normal range. Although the relationship between urinary and dietary calcium in normal subjects is relatively flat, owing to the rather low absorption of dietary calcium, the corresponding slope in idiopathic male calcium-stone formers is much steeper, so that diet plays a critical role in the calcium excretion of this group of calcium-stone formers where recognition of hypercalciuria is particularly important. This intra-individual variation of urinary calcium in stone formers on a free diet is much greater than on a fixed diet and also much greater than in normal subjects on a free diet[10].

The most useful single definition of hypercalciuria is: a calcium excretion of greater than 7.5 mmol/day in women and 10 mmol/day in men, or greater than 0.1 mmol per kg per day in either sex when the patient is screened on a defined 50 mmol daily calcium intake.

CLASSIFICATION

Hypercalciuria may be classified in various ways. A convenient differentiation is to distinguish between primary and secondary hypercalciuria as shown in Table 2.1. Of the secondary hypercalciurias, only the first six conditions are clearly associated with an increased incidence of calcium-stone disease. Primary hyperparathyroidism is

TABLE 2.1 Classification of hypercalciuria

Idiopathic hypercalciuria	*Secondary hypercalciuria*
Absorptive	Primary hyperparathyroidism
Renal	Sarcoidosis
Resorptive	Distal renal tubular acidosis
	Vitamin D excess
	Immobilization
	Medullary sponge kidney
	Acromegaly
	Frusemide therapy
	Thyrotoxicosis
	Glucocortical excess
	Dietary

by far the most important of these causes and has been discussed in detail elsewhere in this book.

Dietary hypercalciuria is important but uncommon. It tends to occur intermittently in a series of urinary collections from a given patient and almost always disappears when the patient is evaluated on a defined diet. Dietary sodium, carbohydrate and phosphate all increase calcium excretion but their influence is relatively minor. High calcium intake itself is a rare cause of hypercalciuria as intake must be extremely high (above 50 mmol/day) if calcium absorption is normal. Protein intake has a more striking effect but can usually be excluded by taking a careful clinical history.

A more satisfactory way to classify hypercalciuria is on a functional basis. There are relatively few fundamental mechanisms which can lead to hypercalciuria:

(1) A defect in renal tubular reabsorption,
(2) An increase in net intestinal calcium absorption,
(3) An increase in bone resorption, or
(4) A combination of these processes.

The two key variables determining the rate of calcium excretion are the filtered load of calcium throughout the day and the efficiency of renal tubular calcium reabsorption. The quantity of calcium excretion in the urine must ultimately be derived from dietary calcium or bone mineral or both. Using this functional classification, idiopathic hypercalciuria can be divided into absorptive, renal and resorptive types.

Absorptive hypercalciuria

This is the commonest cause of absolute hypercalciuria and is characterized by a raised urinary calcium when dietary calcium is normal, which falls when calcium intake is reduced. Calcium absorption is increased and tubular reabsorption of calcium is normal. The hyperabsorption leads to postprandial increases in extracellular calcium concentration, resulting in suppression of parathyroid hormone. Hypercalciuria results from a high load of calcium filtered by the glomeruli. The reduced reabsorption of calcium from the low levels of parathyroid hormone acting on the distal tubule adds a renal component to the net hypercalciuria in this disorder. The excessive renal loss of calcium compensates for the high calcium absorption and maintains the serum concentration of calcium within the normal range.

There is evidence that at least three primary mechanisms may produce this hyperabsorption of calcium. Some of these patients have increased circulating levels of $1,25(OH)_2D_3$ in the absence of hypophosphataemia. These patients may have a primary increase in $1,25(OH)_2D_3$ due to increased sensitivity of renal hydroxy D_3 1α-hydroxylase to the effect of parathyroid hormone[23]. A second group who have intestinal hyperabsorption of calcium have normal plasma concentrations of both phosphate and $1,25(OH)_2D_3$. Such patients have increased intestinal sensitivity to $1,25(OH)_2D_3$ or, possibly, an innate lowering of the intestinal permeability to calcium[24]. Many patients with absorptive hypercalciuria have a primary renal tubular phosphate leak. This leads to reduced plasma phosphate concentration and results in a secondary increase in $1,25(OH)_2D_3$ synthesis. The high circulating levels of this hormone cause increased intestinal calcium absorption resulting in secondary hypoparathyroidism and hypercalciuria[25,26].

Absorptive hypercalciuria contributes substantially to the hypercalciuria of primary hyperparathyroidism, vitamin D poisoning or sarcoidosis, though, in all these conditions, some increase in bone resorption may also be present.

Renal hypercalciuria

Renal hypercalciuria is characterized by a primary defect in renal tubular calcium reabsorption[27,28]. The site of this defect is likely to be the distal nephron. The tubular losses of calcium lead to a slight reduction in plasma calcium, an effect which stimulates the parathyroid glands. Secondary hyperparathyroidism leads to a reduction in plasma phosphate concentration which is a potent stimulant to increased production of $1,25(OH)_2D_3$. Thus, in these patients, increased absorption and urinary excretion of calcium takes place at a low, or low-normal plasma calcium concentration. Histomorphometric findings in these patients reveal a typical pattern of early hyperparathyroidism in bone.

Resorptive hypercalciuria

Patients with resorptive hypercalciuria have a disorder associated with an increased rate of resorption of bone mineral. If net bone resorption (the difference between the rate of bone resorption and mineralization) is sufficiently high, absolute hypercalciuria may ensue. By far the commonest cause of this condition is primary hyperparathyroidism. However, in recent years, the condition of subtle hyperparathyroidism with intermittent hypercalcaemia has been recognized, this condition often presenting with renal stones and resorptive hypercalciuria[29]. The primary abnormality is excess secretion of parathyroid hormone, leading to increased osteoclastic resorption of bone. Intestinal calcium absorption may be increased secondarily by the parathyroid hormone-dependent stimulation of the renal synthesis of $1,25(OH)_2D_3$. Hypercalciuria often occurs since the increase in the filtered load of calcium and the suppressive effect of hypercalcaemia on renal tubular reabsorption of calcium usually overcome the opposing effect of parathyroid hormone enhancing renal calcium reabsorption. Therefore, hypercalciuria is primarily resorptive and secondarily absorptive[30]. Other conditions, such as distal renal tubular acidosis, immobilization and thyrotoxicosis, cause increased mobilization of calcium into the extracellular pool. This results in suppression of parathyroid hormone secretion and $1,25(OH)_2D_3$ synthesis. Calcium absorption in these conditions is decreased but the rise in extracellular calcium concentration leads to increased renal filtering of calcium and hypercalciuria.

The pathophysiological features of the subtypes of idiopathic hypercalciuria are shown in Table 2.2. Although there are many points of similarity between the various subtypes, there are also distinctive differences which form the basis of differential diagnosis.

DIAGNOSTIC TESTS TO DIFFERENTIATE SUBTYPES OF HYPERCALCIURIA

The presence and degree of hypercalciuria should be documented by two or more 24 h urine collections performed on a high-normal (approximately 50 mmol) calcium intake known to contain normal

HYPERCALCIURIA

TABLE 2.2 Pathophysiological features of subtypes of hypercalciuria

Subtype	Calcium absorption	Serum calcium	Urinary calcium	Serum phosphate	Serum 1,25(OH)$_2$D$_3$	Serum PTH	Bone resorption
Absorptive hypercalciuria							
1,25 (OH)$_2$D$_3$	High	Normal	High	Normal	High*	Normal/low	Normal/high
Intestinal	High*	Normal	High	Normal	Normal	Low	Normal
Phosphate leak	High	Normal	High	Low*	High	Normal/low	Normal/high
Renal hypercalciuria	High	Normal/low	High*	Low	High	High	High
Resorptive hypercalciuria							
Primary hyperparathyroidism	High	High/normal	High	Low	High	High*	High
Other causes	Low	Normal	High	Normal	Low	Low	High*

* primary abnormality

43

quantities of protein (about 1 g/kg body weight) and sodium (about 100 mmol/day). It is important to screen stone formers while taking an unrestricted calcium intake because an increase in intestinal calcium absorption is common to each of the major subgroups of idiopathic hypercalciuria. The diagnosis of secondary hypercalciuria is important and is usually straightforward, from history, physical examination and routine clinical tests. Dietary hypercalciuria is identified by careful dietary history and the demonstration that alteration in the diet brings the excess calcium excretion into the normal range.

The diagnosis of idiopathic hypercalciuria is achieved by exclusion of the secondary causes. The principal aim of further investigation in idiopathic hypercalciuria is to differentiate between the various subtypes. No approach to this differential diagnosis has received universal acceptance. Indeed, criteria for diagnosis vary considerably between different investigators, as do reported incidence figures for the frequency of the various hypercalciuric subtypes in their patients. However, there is a growing consensus that patients with absorptive hypercalciuria constitute the clear majority of patients with idiopathic hypercalciuria.

Formerly, the tests required to differentiate these causes were sophisticated and the patients required admission to a metabolic ward for careful dietary calcium adjustment and detailed collections of blood and urine over several days. However, a single calcium load study has been devised that can be performed easily on outpatients[28,31]. Various modifications have been suggested but the original protocol remains satisfactory for most uses. The test makes several basic assumptions:

(a) During fasting, urinary calcium is raised in renal hypercalciuria or resorptive hypercalciuria.
(b) After an oral calcium load, urinary calcium rises in absorptive hypercalciuria.
(c) Urinary cyclic adenosine monophosphate, after a calcium load, provides a reliable measure of parathyroid hormone activity.

The patient is placed on a low calcium diet of 10 mmol/day for the previous seven days. The test is a six-hour study after an overnight fast. From 9 pm on the evening before the test, the patient is fasted and only allowed to drink distilled water. On the morning of the test, urine is collected for two hours while fasting and then for four hours after ingestion of 50 mmol of calcium mixed in a synthetic meal. The samples are analysed for calcium, creatinine and cyclic adenosine monophosphate. At the beginning of the test, 600 ml distilled water are ingested, followed by 300 ml at the time of the synthetic meal and 300 ml midway through the next 4 h.

The rationale for this test is as follows: a patient with a high excretion rate of calcium whilst fasting may have either a renal leak of calcium or hypercalciuria secondary to bone resorption. These two possibilities can be differentiated by a serum calcium level which will be normal or low in cases of renal leak or high in cases of hyperparathyroidism. The extent of renal calcium excretion following an oral load of calcium provides an indirect assessment of intestinal calcium absorption.

This test was designed to differentiate between the two major forms of idiopathic hypercalciuria. Fasting urinary calcium and cyclic adenosine monophosphate are increased in patients with renal hypercalciuria, because of the renal leak of calcium, and in those with secondary hyperparathyroidism. In cases of absorptive hypercalciuria, these values are within the normal range but there is an exaggerated urinary calcium excretion following an oral calcium load, reflecting an enhanced intestinal absorption of calcium. It is important that the patient is adequately prepared before this test with a low-calcium low-sodium diet. Without this preparation, patients with intestinal hyperabsorption of calcium may have abnormally high values of fasting urinary calcium.

Absorptive hypercalciuria is diagnosed by the combination of hypercalciuria and suppressed cyclic adenosine monophosphate excretion, a rise occurring in urinary calcium excretion after a calcium load.

Renal hypercalciuria is diagnosed by a combination of hypercalciuria and increased cyclic adenosine monophosphate excretion on a restricted calcium intake, the high-dose calcium load causing an increase in urinary calcium and a suppression of urinary cyclic adenosine monophosphate to normal.

In patients with resorptive hypercalciuria, the calcium load induces hypercalcaemia with inappropriate partial suppression of parathyroid function.

Other more simple tests have been designed to differentiate absorptive from renal hypercalciuria[27]. Patients are treated with a 10 mmol/day calcium diet for 13 days. On the first six days, 500 mg supplemental calcium carbonate are added to increase the total calcium intake to 22.5 mmol/day. Twenty-four-hour urine collections are made on days 5 and 6 at the end of the high-calcium intake, and days 12 and 13 at the end of the low-calcium intake. This test confirms, in a straightforward simple manner, the presence or absence of hypercalciuria and suggests absorptive hypercalciuria if there is a significant fall in urinary calcium excretion at the end of the period on a low-calcium diet.

A further test[32] which may be helpful in differentiating resorptive hypercalciuria compares the urinary calcium excretion during a two-hour period in the morning following an overnight fast and subsequently the following day after the administration of 20 g sodium cellulose phosphate as an oral calcium-binding agent. In normal subjects and patients with absorptive and renal hypercalciuria, calcium excretion falls. However, in patients with hypercalciuria, whose calcium excretion does not fall following cellulose phosphate, a resorptive cause for hypercalciuria can usually be identified.

SUMMARY OF DIAGNOSTIC CRITERIA

The features which differentiate the subtypes of hypercalciuria are shown in Table 2.2.

Absorptive hypercalciuria type 1 is characterized by:

(1) Normal plasma calcium,
(2) Normal fasting urinary calcium,
(3) Exaggerated urinary calcium following an oral calcium load,
(4) Normal or suppressed parathyroid function,
(5) Urinary calcium, on 10 mmol per day calcium diet, >5 mmol per day.

Absorptive hypercalciuria type 2 is characterized by the same biochemical features as type 1 except for normal urinary calcium on a restricted diet.

Renal hypercalciuria is characterized by:

(1) Normal plasma calcium,

(2) High fasting urinary calcium,
(3) Secondary hyperparathyroidism.

Primary hyperparathyroidism is characterized by:

(1) Hypercalcaemia,
(2) Hypophosphataemia,
(3) Hypercalciuria,
(4) Increased or inappropriately high serum PTH.

TREATMENT

Patients with hypercalciuria who form recurrent urinary calculi composed of calcium oxalate or phosphate can face a lifetime of recurrent pain. Many treatments have been postulated but there is often conflicting evidence for their efficacy. In prospective studies, the degree of hypercalciuria did not predict the risk of stone recurrence[33] or the efficacy of treatments which decreased urinary calcium[34-36]. Without treatment, recurrence is likely in only 7% of patients per year and is even less common in older men and patients without renal calcification[33,37].

Fluid intake

The simplest way to reduce the urinary concentration of calcium is to increase urinary volume. A fluid intake sufficient to produce a urinary volume of 2.5 L is often advised, but it is very difficult to drink more than 3 L/day. By increasing urine output, urinary concentration of ions and the saturation of stone-forming salts are lowered. The intake of fluid should be distributed throughout the day to ensure a constantly high urine output, and, since the concentration of urine increases during the night, a pint of water should be taken before retiring at bedtime. During heavy exercise or in hot weather, fluid intake should be increased further.

Objective evidence that a high fluid intake reduces stone formation is scarce, though *in vitro* studies have confirmed a reduction in crystallization of calcium salts following urinary dilution[38]. Biochemical studies show that the risk of stone formation increases markedly as urine volume falls below 1200 ml per day[39]. This observation is supported by data from a study of desert dwellers in Israel, showing that the prevalence of stone disease was inversely related to urine volume[40]. In a study of stone formers advised to pass at least 2.5 L urine a day, those who seemed to stop forming stones had achieved higher urine volumes than the other patients[37].

Dietary manipulation

Calcium restriction

Dietary calcium restriction of less than 10 mmol/day is ill advised, even in patients with absorptive hypercalciuria as negative calcium balance may occur. Restriction of dietary calcium intake over long periods is difficult to maintain and the long-term results are not encouraging[41]. However, moderate calcium restriction of 10–15 mmol/day may be useful in absorptive hypercalciuria since this dietary change alone may be sufficient to control the hypercalciuria, or may enable reduced dosage of other medication to be used.

Calcium restriction is neither necessary nor indicated in patients with normal intestinal absorption of calcium. However, excessive intake of calcium, greater than 50 mmol/day, should be avoided in these patients since this high intake may further increase hypercalciuria.

Sodium restriction

A high sodium intake may contribute to calcium-stone formation by augmenting renal excretion of calcium, thereby inducing secondary hyperparathyroidism. To overcome this effect, moderate sodium restriction of around 100 mmol/day may be helpful in all patients with idiopathic hypercalciuria.

Dietary protein

Excessive ingestion of foods rich in animal proteins enhances calcium excretion. The institution of a vegetarian diet may induce other alterations in the urine, including increased oxalate excretion, and may oppose the beneficial effects of reduced calcium and uric acid excretion[42]. It would, therefore, seem sensible to eliminate dietary excesses of protein in patients with idiopathic hypercalciuria.

Dietary fibre

The ideal therapeutic treatment for patients with idiopathic hypercalciuria, many of whom will not develop recurrence of renal stones, is one which is easily taken, inexpensive, free from side effects and requires little medical supervision. Dietary fibre fulfils all these criteria. Thirty years ago, it was shown that a significant reduction in urinary calcium excretion could be produced in patients with idiopathic hypercalciuria when treated with sodium phytate[4]. More recently the same effect has been shown to occur with a high-fibre diet[43], the effect being the result of precipitation of calcium phytate in the intestine. Further studies have shown that urinary calcium excretion was reduced in 86% of patients who took 24 g of fine unprocessed bran daily in divided doses[44]. In addition, wheat bran has been shown to oppose the increased calcium absorption rate following glucose loading.

Drug therapy

Thiazide diuretics

It has been known for many years that thiazide diuretic drugs lower the urinary calcium of both normocalciuric and hypercalciuric patients[45]. Thiazides act by stimulating calcium reabsorption from the distal convoluted tubule. Thiazides also enhance sodium excretion, leading to a reduced extracellular fluid volume. A reduced glomerular filtration rate will follow and this leads to a fall in the filtered load of calcium, resulting in an increase in fractional calcium reabsorption and a fall in urinary calcium. Extracellular fluid volume depletion may contribute to the hypercalciuric effect as thiazides been shown to lower calcium more promptly if extracellular fluid volume is reduced before their administration. However, in balance studies, the peak fall in urinary calcium output occurred between the third and ninth day after the onset of treatment, well after the peak of sodium diuresis which was usually seen within 36 h.

Thiazide diuretics have a variable effect on intestinal calcium absorption. In patients with absorptive hypercalciuria, intestinal hyperabsorption of calcium persists despite restoration of a normal urinary calcium[46,47]. However, in patients with renal hypercalciuria, thiazides cause a significant decrease in intestinal calcium absorption, resulting from the correction of the renal leak of calcium and thereby removing the parathyroid stimulus to increased production of $1,25(OH)_2D_3$[46,47]. In such patients, a significant fall in serum concentration of $1,25(OH)_2D_3$ has been demonstrated[46].

Many studies have shown that the recurrence rate of stone formation is reduced by approximately half by the long-term use of thiazide diuretics. However, controlled trials are few. Several short trials have failed to show a benefit from hydrochlorothiazide[36] or bendroflumethiazide[48], though a controlled trial lasting 3 years did show a benefit which would have been missed had the trial been shorter[33]. Prolonged treatment is therefore promising for hypercalciuric stone formers. However, the long-term effects of thiazides may prove troublesome in some patients. Should potassium supplements prove necessary, potassium citrate is a more appropriate treatment for stone formers than potassium chloride. Citrate is an inhibitor of the formation of calcium-containing renal stones as it reduces the saturation of stone-forming calcium salts by forming a soluble complex with calcium[49]. In addition, citrate may inhibit the crystal growth of calcium phosphate[50,51] and calcium oxalate[52,53]. Thiazide therapy is complicated by hypercalciuria, a consequence of hypokalaemia. Both these abnormalities are corrected by oral potassium citrate[54].

Sodium cellulose phosphate

Sodium cellulose phosphate, the sodium salt of the phosphoric ester of cellulose, is an ion exchange cellulose with special affinity for divalent cations, the result of the configuration of the phosphate radicals attached to the cellulose molecule. In the stomach, it exchanges sodium for calcium which is eliminated in the faeces, thus preventing the absorption of dietary calcium[55]. Similarly, it binds with secreted calcium preventing its reabsorption. The diminution in calcium absorption is accompanied by a reduction in the renal excretion of calcium and a slight increase in urinary phosphates. The major theoretical drawback to this treatment is a reciprocal increase in urinary oxalate excretion, the benefit of the hypocalciuria being offset by hyperoxaluria. It may also lower the urinary excretion of magnesium from intestinal binding of magnesium. Thus, the apparent solubility of the principal stone constituent in urine (calcium oxalate) may be reduced because less oxalate would be complexed by magnesium. There have been a few studies which have claimed a reduction in stone formation in hypercalciuric patients treated with sodium cellulose phosphate[56,57]. These have advised caution concerning drug dosage, a reduction in dietary oxalate and magnesium supplements. Cellulose phosphate treatment may further exaggerate secondary hyperparathyroidism in patients with renal hypercalciuria. Thus, the use of this drug should be restricted to patients with absorptive hypercalciuria not controlled on moderate calcium restriction alone. As calcium load tests and parathyroid hormone assays may not be readily available for regular clinical use, cellulose phosphate cannot be recommended for indiscriminate therapy.

Orthophosphates

Orthophosphate treatment of patients with idiopathic hypercalciuria reduces the urinary excretion of calcium and increases inhibitory activity by raising urinary pyrophosphate[58,59]. These effects result in a significant reduction in the frequency of passage of large crystals and aggregates of calcium oxalate in urine. Studies have shown varying clinical success with this form of treatment[58–60].

Orthophosphate salts are available as potassium acid phosphate, neutral mixtures consisting of potassium and sodium phosphates or potassium phosphates alone, or an alkaline mixture consisting of disodium and dipotassium phosphates. One possible explanation for the differing results of this therapy is provided by evidence that the acid load in certain of these preparations may have had a deleterious effect on calcium and citrate metabolism[61]. Diarrhoea may be an occasional problem, particularly in patients with gastrointestinal disorders. Sodium-containing mixtures may be unsuitable for hypertensive patients for whom neutral mixtures of potassium phosphates are preferable.

Diphosphonates

Diphosphonates (e.g. etidronate disodium (Didronal)) are analogues of naturally occurring inhibitor pyrophosphates. They are potent inhibitors of the formation and aggregation of crystalline calcium phosphate or calcium oxalate and have been reported to be effective in decreasing calculus formation in experimental animals[62]. Unfortunately, in man, they cause a secondary rise in oxalate absorption and urinary excretion, which, in most instances, negates the beneficial effect on inhibitory activity. In addition, the high doses used in man may produce significant changes in bone mineralization[63]. Thus, at present, diphosphonates hold little promise for the treatment of hypercalciuric stone disease.

Medical management of patients with hypercalciuria

Medical management of patients with renal stone disease involves determination of the chemical composition of the stone, identification of the predisposing chemical abnormality in the urine, searching for a predisposing disease which may be present, alteration in diet, drug therapy and subsequent monitoring of the activity of the stone-forming process by radiological, clinical and laboratory means to ascertain the effectiveness of treatment. Many physicians regard thiazide diuretics as the treatment of choice for idiopathic hypercalciuria and question the necessity of subclassifying hypercalciuric patients into renal and absorptive subgroups. However, the rapid progress made in renal stone research to elucidate these subgroups has led to the possibility of a selective treatment approach for hypercalciuria[50,64]. The advantages of such an approach are that the treatment corrects physicochemical abnormalities in the urine, overcomes physiological derangements in patients with stones, inhibits stone formation, does not cause significant side effects and prevents extrarenal manifestations of the disease process. On the basis of current knowledge of the aetiology of hypercalciuria, six treatments may be considered to satisfy the criteria for selective treatment since they have been shown to reverse much of the physicochemical and physiological derangements underlying the given cause of the stone formation.

(1) Sodium cellulose phosphate for absorptive hypercalciuria type 1

Sodium cellulose phosphate 10–15 g/day, may be used to control absorptive hypercalciuria since it has been shown to correct the intestinal hyperabsorption of calcium by binding calcium into the intestinal tract. It has been reported to restore the normal physicochemical environment of urine by reducing saturation of urine with respect to brushite ($CaHPO_4.2H_2O$). However, the treatment may cause secondary hyperoxaluria and reduced magnesium excretion. Therefore, it is usual to combine cellulose phosphate treatment with moderate oxalate restriction and to provide oral magnesium supplements in the form of magnesium gluconate, 1–1.5 g b.d., separately from the cellulose phosphate.

(2) Thiazides for absorptive hypercalciuria type 1

Thiazide diuretics in the form of hydrochlorothiazide, 50 mg b.d., may not be ideally indicated for absorptive hypercalciuria since they do not restore normal calcium absorption. However, this treatment is a reasonable alternative to sodium cellulose phosphate. Thiazides have been shown to correct hypercalciuria, reduce urinary saturation and enhance inhibitor activity against spontaneous nucleation of both calcium oxalate and brushite. As hypocitraturia may develop, particularly when hypokalaemia is present, it may be necessary to add potassium supplements even in the absence of symptomatic hypokalaemia.

(3) Thiazides for renal hypercalciuria

Thiazides represent an ideal treatment for renal hypercalciuria since they correct the renal leak of calcium, thereby restoring parathyroid function, serum $1,25(OH)_2D_3$ and calcium absorption to normal.

(4) Orthophosphates for hypophosphataemic absorptive hypercalciuria

Orthophosphate treatment in the form of a neutral salt of sodium and potassium providing 1.5 g phosphorus in three divided doses daily is a logical treatment, as raising plasma phosphate results in inhibition of $1,25(OH)_2D_3$ synthesis. This treatment has also been shown to reduce urinary saturation of calcium oxalate and to inhibit spontaneous nucleation of brushite and calcium oxalate.

(5) Thiazides and allopurinol for absorptive hypercalciuria with hyperuricosuria

If hypercalciuria coexists with hyperuricosuria, it is reasonable to speculate that both these abnormalities contribute to stone formation. Combined treatment with thiazides and allopurinol should lower both urinary calcium and uric acid, thereby reducing stone formation.

(6) High fluid intake and low calcium diet for absorptive hypercalciuria type 2

Certain patients with absorptive hypercalciuria have a less severe form of the condition, absorption and renal excretion of calcium being normal during a low calcium intake, though elevated during an increased intake of calcium. A low calcium intake of 10–15 mmol/day and high fluid intake, sufficient to achieve a minimum urinary output of 2–2.5 L/day is indicated since normocalciuria can be restored by dietary calcium restriction alone and increased urinary volume has been shown to reduce urinary saturation of calcium oxalate.

References

1. Flocks, R. H. (1939). Calcium and phosphorus excretion in the urine of patients with renal or ureteral calculi. *J. Am. Med. Assoc.*, **113**, 1466–71
2. Flocks, R. H. (1940). Calcium urolithiasis: the role of calcium and metabolism in the pathogenesis and treatment of calcium urolithiasis. *J. Urol. (Baltimore)*, **43**, 214–33
3. Albright, F., Henneman, P., Benedict, P. H. and Forbes, A. P. (1953). Idiopathic hypercalciuria. *Proc. R. Soc. Med.*, **46**, 1077–81
4. Henneman, P. H., Benedict, P. H., Forbes, A. P. and Dudley, H. R. (1958). Idiopathic hypercalciuria: importance of dietary calcium in the definition of hypercalciuria. *N. Engl. J. Med.*, **259**, 802–7
5. Jackson, W. P. U. and Dancaster, C. (1959). A consideration of the hypercalciuria in sarcoidosis, idiopathic hypercalciuria and that produced by vitamin D. A new suggestion regarding calcium metabolism. *J. Clin. Endocrinol. Metab.*, **19**, 658–80
6. Mehes, K. and Szelid, Z. (1980). Autosomal dominant inheritance of hypercalciuria. *Eur. J. Paediatr.*, **133**, 239–42
7. Sutton, R. A. L. and Dirks, J. H. (1978). Renal handling of calcium. *Fed. Proc.*, **37**, 2112–19
8. Costanzo, L. S. and Windhager, E. E. (1980). Effects of PTH, ADH and cyclic AMP on distal tubular Ca and Na reabsorption. *Am. J. Physiol.*, **239**, f478–85
9. Shareghi, G. R. and Stoner, L. C. (1978). Calcium transport across segments of the rabbit distal nephron in vitro. *Am. J. Physiol.*, **235**, f367–75
10. Broadus, A. E. and Thier, S. O. (1979). The metabolic basis of renal stone disease. *N. Engl. J. Med.*, **300**, 839–45
11. Robertson, W. G., Peacock, M., Marshall, D. H. and Speed, R. (1981). The prevalence of urinary stone disease in practising vegetarians. *Fortschr. Urol. Nephrol.*, **17**, 6–14
12. Lemann, J., Adams, N. D. and Gray, R. W. (1979). Urinary calcium excretion in human beings. *N. Engl. J. Med.*, **301**, 535–41
13. Whiting, S. J. and Draper, H. H. (1980). The role of sulphate in the calciuria of high protein diet in the rat. *J. Nutr.*, **110**, 212–22

14. Linkswiler, H. M., Joyce, C. L. and Arnaud, C. R. (1974). Calcium retention of young adult males as affected by level of protein and of calcium intake. *Trans. N.Y. Acad. Sci.*, **36**, 333–40
15. Goldfarb, S., Westby, G. R., Goldberg, M. and Agus, Z. S. (1977). Renal tubular effects of chronic phosphate depletion. *J. Clin. Invest.*, **59**, 770–8
16. Dominguez, J. H., Gray, R. W. and Lemann, J. Jr. (1976). Dietary phosphate deprivation in women and men: effects on mineral and acid balances, parathyroid hormone and the metabolism of 25(OH) vitamin D. *J. Clin. Endocrinol. Metab.*, **43**, 1056–68
17. Lemann, J. Jr., Lennon, E. J., Piering, W. R., Prien, E. L. Jr. and Ricanati, E. S. (1970). Evidence that glucose ingestion inhibits net renal tubular reabsorption of calcium and magnesium in man. *J. Lab. Clin. Med.*, **75**, 578–85
18. Sutton, R. A. L., Wong, N. L. M. and Dirks, J. H. (1979). Effects of metabolic acidosis and alkalosis on sodium and calcium transport in the dog kidney. *Kidney Int.*, **15**, 520–33
19. Batlle, D. C., Itsarayounguen, K., Hays, S., Arruda, J. A. L. and Kurtzman, N. A. (1982). Parathyroid hormone is not anticalciuric during chronic metabolic acidosis. *Kidney Int.*, **22**, 264–71
20. Peraino, R. A. and Suki, W. N. (1980). Urine HCO_3^- augments renal Ca^{++} absorption independent of systemic acid based changes. *Am. J. Physiol.*, **238**, f394–8
21. Robertson, W. G., Gallagher, J. C., Marshall, D. H., Peacock, M. and Nordin, B. E. C. (1974). Seasonal variations in urinary excretion of calcium. *Br. Med. J.*, **41**, 436–7
22. Robertson, W. G. and Morgan D. B. (1972). The distribution of urinary calcium excretions in normal persons and stone formers. *Clin. Chim. Acta*, **37**, 503–8
23. Evans, R. A., Hills, E., Wong, S. Y. P., Wyndham, L. E., Eade, Y. and Dunstan, C. R. (1984). The pathogenesis of idiopathic hypercalciuria: evidence for parathyroid hyperfunction. *Q. J. Med.*, **53**, 41–53
24. Stanbury, S. W. (1980). Idiopathic hypercalciuria (absorptive hypercalciuria). In Norman, A. W. (ed.) *Vitamin D: Molecular Biology and Clinical Nutrition*, pp. 300–2. (New York: Marcel Dekker)
25. Shen, F. H., Baylink, D. J., Nielsen, R. L., Sherrard, D. J., Ivey, J. L. and Haussler, M. R. (1977). Increased serum 1,25-dihydroxy vitamin D in idiopathic hypercalciuria. *J. Lab. Clin. Med.*, **90**, 955–62
26. Gray, R. W., Wilz, D. R., Caldas, A. E. and Lemann, J. (1977). The importance of phosphate in regulating plasma 1,25-$(OH)_2$-vitamin D levels in humans: studies in healthy subjects, in calcium-stone formers and in patients with primary hyperparathyroidism. *J. Clin. Endocrinol. Metab.*, **45**, 299–306
27. Broadus, A. E., Dominguez, M. and Bartter, F. C. (1978). Pathophysiological studies in idiopathic hypercalciuria: use of an oral calcium tolerance test to characterise distinctive hypercalciuric groups. *J. Clin. Endocrinol. Metab.*, **47**, 751–60
28. Pak, C. Y. C., Britton, F., Peterson, R., Ward, D., Northcutt, C., Breslau, N. A., McGuire, J., Sakhaee, K., Bush, S., Nicar, M., Norman, D. A. and Peters, P. (1980). Ambulatory evaluation of nephrolithiasis. *Am. J. Med.*, **69**, 19–30
29. Broadus, A. E., Horst, R. L., Littledike, E. T., Mahaffey, J. E. and Rasmussen, H. (1980). Primary hyperparathyroidism with intermittent hypercalcaemia: serial observations and simple diagnosis by means of an oral calcium tolerance test. *Clin. Endocrinol.*, **12**, 225–35

30. Broadus, A. E., Horst, R. L., Lang, R., Littledike, E. T. and Rasmussen, H. (1980). The importance of circulating 1,25-dihydroxy vitamin D in the pathogenesis of hypercalciuria and renal stone formation in primary hyperparathyroidism. *N. Engl. J. Med.*, **302**, 421–6
31. Pak, C. Y. C., Kaplan, R., Bone, H., Townsend, J. and Waters, O. (1975). A simple test for the diagnosis of absorptive, resorptive and renal hypercalciurias. *N. Engl. J. Med.*, **292**, 497–500
32. Tschöpe, W. and Ritz, E. (1985). Hypercalciuria and nephrolithiasis. *Contr. Nephrol.*, **49**, 94–103
33. Marshall, V., White, R. H., Chaput de Saintonge, D. M., Tresidder, G. C. and Blandy, J. P. (1975). The natural history of renal and ureteric calculi. *Br. J. Urol.*, **47**, 117–24
34. Laerum, E. and Larsen, S. (1984). Thiazide prophylaxis of urolithiasis: a double-blind study in general practice. *Acta Med. Scand.*, **215**, 383–9
35. Backman, U., Danielson, B. G., Johansson, S., Ljunghall, S. and Wilkström, B. (1979). Effects of therapy with bendroflumethiazide in patients with recurrent renal calcium stones. *Br. J. Urol.*, **51**, 175–80
36. Scholz, D., Schwille, P. O. and Sigel, A. (1982). Double-blind study with thiazide in recurrent calcium lithiasis. *J. Urol.*, **128**, 903–7
37. Ettinger, B. (1979). Recurrence of nephrolithiasis. A six-year prospective study. *Am. J. Med.*, **67**, 245–8
38. Pak, C. Y. C., Sakhaee, K., Crowther, C. and Brinkley, L. (1980). Evidence justifying a high fluid intake in treatment of nephrolithiasis. *Ann. Intern. Med.*, **93**, 36–9
39. Robertson, W. G., Peacock, M., Heyburn, P. J. and Hanes, F. A. (1980). Epidemiological risk factors in calcium stone disease. *Scand. J. Urol. Nephrol. (Suppl.)*, **53**, 15–28
40. Frank, M. and De Vries, A. (1966). Prevention of urolithiasis. *Arch. Environ. Health*, **13**, 625–30
41. Baker, L. R. I. and Mallinson, W. J. W. (1979). Dietary treatment of idiopathic hypercalciuria. *Br. J. Urol.*, **51**, 181–3
42. Brockis, J. G., Levitt, A. J. and Cruthers, S. M. (1982). The effects of vegetable and animal protein diets on calcium, urate and oxalate excretion. *Br. J. Urol.*, **54**, 590–3
43. Heaton, K. W. and Pomare, E. W. (1974). Effect of bran on blood lipids and calcium. *Lancet*, **1**, 49–50
44. Shah, P. J. R., Williams, G. and Green, N. A. (1980). Idiopathic hypercalciuria: its control with unprocessed bran. *Br. J. Urol.*, **52**, 426–9
45. Yendt, E. R. and Cohanim, M. (1978). Thiazides in calcium urolithiasis. *Can. Med. Assoc. J.*, **118**, 755–8
46. Zerwekh, J. E. and Pak, C. Y. C. (1980). Selective effects of thiazide therapy on serum 1α, 25-dihydroxy vitamin D and intestinal calcium absorption in renal absorptive hypercalciurias. *Metabolism*, **29**, 13–17
47. Barilla, D. E., Tolentino, R., Kaplan, R. A. and Pak, C. Y. C. (1978). Selective effects of thiazide on intestinal absorption of calcium in absorptive and renal hypercalciurias. *Metabolism*, **27**, 125–31
48. Brocks, P., Dahl, C., Wolf, H. and Transbøl, I. (1981). Do thiazides prevent recurrent idiopathic renal calcium stones? *Lancet*, **2**, 124–5
49. Pak, C. Y. C., Nicar, M. and Northcutt, C. (1982). The definition of the mech-

anism of hypercalciuria is necessary for the treatment of recurrent stone formers. *Contrib. Nephrol.*, **33**, 136–51
50. Meyer, J. L. and Thomas, W. C. Jr. (1982). Trace metal–citric acid complexes as inhibitors of calcification and crystal growth. I. Effects of Fe(III), Cr(III), and Al(III) complexes on calcium phosphate crystal growth. *J. Urol.*, **128**, 1372–5
51. Bisaz, S., Felix, R., Neuman, W. and Fleisch, H. (1978). Quantitative determination of inhibitors of calcium phosphate precipitation in whole urine. *Min. Electrolyte Metab.*, **1**, 74–83
52. Meyer, J. L. and Smith, L. H. (1975). Growth of calcium oxalate crystals. II. Inhibition by natural urinary crystal growth inhibitors. *Invest. Urol.*, **13**, 36–9
53. Meyer, J. L. and Thomas, W. C. (1982). Trace metal–citric acid complexes as inhibitors of calcification and crystal growth. II. Effects of Fe(III), Cr(III), and Al(III), complexes on calcium oxalate crystal growth. *J. Urol.*, **128**, 1376–8
54. Nicar, M. J., Peterson, R. and Pak, C. Y. C. (1984). Use of potassium citrate as potassium supplement during thiazide therapy of calcium nephrolithiasis. *J. Urol.*, **131**, 430–3
55. Pak, C. Y. C. (1973). Sodium cellulose phosphate: mechanism of action and effect on mineral metabolism. *J. Clin. Pharmacol.*, **13**, 15–27
56. Backman, U., Danielson, B. G., Johansson, G., Ljunghall, S. and Wikström, B. (1980). Treatment of recurrent calcium stone formation with cellulose phosphate. *J. Urol.*, **123**, 9–13
57. Pak, C. Y. C. (1981). A cautious use of sodium cellulose phosphate in the management of calcium nephrolithiasis. *Invest. Urol.*, **19**, 187–90
58. Fleisch, H., Bisaz, S. and Care, A. D. (1964). Effect of orthophosphates on urinary pyrophosphate excretion and the prevention of urolithiasis. *Lancet*, **1**, 1065–7
59. Thomas, W. C. Jr. (1971). Effectiveness and mode of action of orthophosphates in patients with calcareous renal calculi. *Trans. Am. Clin. Climatol. Assoc.*, **83**, 113–24
60. Ettinger, B. (1976). Recurrent nephrolithiasis: natural history and effect of phosphate therapy. *Am. J. Med.*, **61**, 200–6
61. Lau, K., Wolf, C., Nussbaum, P., Weiner, B., De Oreo, P., Slatopolsky, E., Agus, Z. and Goldfarb, S. (1979). Differing effects of acid versus neutral phosphate therapy of hypercalciuria. *Kidney Int.*, **16**, 736–42
62. Fraser, D., Russell, R. G. G., Pohler, O., Robertson, W. G. and Fleisch, H. (1972). The influence of disodium ethane 1-hydroxy-1,1-diphosphonate (EHDP) on the development of experimentally induced urinary stones in rats. *Clin. Sci. Mol. Med.*, **42**, 197–207
63. Jowsey, J., Riggs, B. L., Kelly, P. J., Hoffman, D. L. and Bordier, P. (1971). The treatment of osteoporosis with disodium ethane-1-hydroxy-1,1-diphosphonate. *J. Lab. Clin. Med.*, **78**, 574–84
64. Pak, C. Y. C., Peters, P., Hurt, G., Kadesky, M., Fine, M., Reisman, D., Splann, F., Caramela, C., Freeman, A., Britton, F., Sakhaee, K. and Breslau, N. (1981). Is selective therapy of recurrent nephrolithiasis possible? *Am. J. Med.*, **71**, 615–22

3
RECURRENT CALCULI

C. A. C. CHARLTON

INTRODUCTION

The prevention of recurrent calculi lies in correcting the single or multiple abnormalities which predispose to the recurrence. In our present state of knowledge, a minority of stone formers can be reassured that all the causative factors have been identified, and that, by taking known appropriate action, the patient can be virtually guaranteed a cure with a minimal chance of further stone formation. This applies in primary hyperparathyroidism, in the relatively rare cystine stone and in the majority of pure uric acid stone formers; but regrettably this is not the case in the largest group of patients with an identifiable abnormality, namely hypercalciuria. In a carefully supervised group of 124 stone formers with idiopathic hypercalciuria[1], the urinary calcium was brought into the normal range, yet over one half continued to develop new or larger calculi. It follows that there must be other unidentified factors which are in part responsible for the continued urolithiasis, and a possible explanation for this is discussed at the end of this chapter.

Calcium stone disease accounts for around 70% of all urinary calculi seen in the Western world. It is clear that six factors are involved in this disorder, namely urine volume and pH, the concentration of the urinary crystalloids calcium, oxalate and uric acid, and the presence and nature of urinary mucopolysaccharides. These have been labelled as the six risk factors in calcium stone disease of the urinary tract[2], and restoration of these factors to normal could be expected to prevent further stone formation. These factors will be further examined. Infected stones account for 10–30% of urinary calculi, and the recurrence rate can be drastically reduced by meticulous surgical clearance (supplemented if necessary by intrarenal irrigation using a stone solvent) and careful bacteriological surveillance.

URIC ACID STONES

There are three correctable factors which lead to the formation of the pure uric acid calculus; these are the concentration of urinary uric acid and the volume and pH of the urine. A fourth factor, ill understood, is the role played by urinary mucopolysaccharides.

About a quarter of patients with uric acid stones have hyperuricosuria. In most of these, an excessive dietary intake of purines is found to be the cause; the foods responsible for this are liver, kidney, sweetbreads, anchovies, sardines and brains; and their dietary intake must be severely restricted. An increase in urinary uric acid is found in some cases of primary or secondary gout, and in those disorders in which there is considerable breakdown of cells with the liberation of nucleic acid, e.g. polycythaemia, leukaemia and during cytotoxic chemotherapy. Nucleic acid is metabolized through a series of intermediate compounds to xanthine and hypoxanthine, which, in turn, are converted to uric acid as a result of the action of xanthine oxidase. This enzyme is inhibited by allopurinol, which thus prevents a rise in the serum and urinary uric acid concentrations. The occasional side effects of this drug include a mild rash and dyspepsia, but it may also precipitate an acute attack of gout (probably due to tophi going into solution as a result of the fall in serum and tissue uric acid levels). It is therefore advisable to start therapy at a daily dose of 100 mg, increasing at weekly intervals until the serum uric acid level is brought back into the normal range.

Uric acid excretion also occurs in the distal ileum, and those patients with ulcerative colitis and Crohn's disease who have an ileostomy will excrete increased amounts of uric acid in their urine. Furthermore, an ileostomy results in considerable fluid losses, including alkaline digestive juices, which in turn cause a decreased urine volume and an acid urine, both of which are risk factors in the formation of uric acid stones.

The urinary pH is a critical factor in determining the solubility product of uric acid and thus the spontaneous nucleation of crystals. At a pH of 5.35, one half of all urinary urate is in the undissociated, less soluble form of uric acid; if the pH is raised to 6.5, less than one sixth of the total urinary urates exist in this undissociated form, which is then below the solubility product for uric acid. Hence, alkalis in the form of 6–8 g potassium citrate should be ingested daily. If the sodium salt is given, care must be taken to avoid congestive cardiac failure and hypertension. The patient should monitor the urinary pH with litmus paper, aiming at a pH of 6.5–7.0. In some cases, it may also be necessary to add sodium bicarbonate to achieve this objective. Similarly, patients should monitor the urine output, ensuring they drink enough to excrete 2.5 L urine a day.

The role of urinary mucopolysaccharides in stone formation is by no means clear, and it is probably misleading to think of these substances as inhibitors of crystallization. It is more logical to think of these macromolecules in terms of size. For a given volume of these substances, the smaller the aggregates, the greater the surface area available for the adsorption of uric acid and urates; the latter are thus taken 'out of solution' and this both reduces the concentration of the crystalloids and prevents supersaturation and crystallization (see later).

THE INFECTED STONE

The struvite or magnesium ammonium phosphate stone is only found in an infected urinary tract. The infecting organisms are urea-splitting bacteria, commonly of the proteus variety, which cause the production of ammonia; an alkaline urine is consequently invariably present. Magnesium ammonium phosphate becomes increasingly insoluble in alkaline urine, and supersaturation occurs with resulting spontaneous crystalluria. The formation product of calcium phosphate is lower than that of magnesium phosphate and hence the former compound often forms a major component of these infected stones. The infecting organisms are incorporated into the substance of the stone, making it physically impossible for the antibiotics in the surrounding urine to percolate into the inner reaches of the stone. Consequently, although the urine may be sterile, as a result of appropriate antibiotic administration, this is suppressive chemotherapy only. On withdrawal of the antibiotic, the organisms will reappear in the urine within days as they multiply within the confines of the stone, pass on to its surface and so into the urine.

To prevent further calculus formation, the stones must therefore be completely cleared from the urinary collecting system. In this context, it must be remembered that it is not unusual to find a soft unmineralized matrix (soft pultaceous material) adjacent to and continuous with a well-mineralized component, the latter being recognized as the calculus on X-ray. It seems likely that the matrix (translucent to X-ray) is the precursor of the stone, and occupies the collecting system to form the subsequent staghorn calculus. Until recently, removal of a stone involved open surgery and, when incision of the renal parenchyma was indicated because the stones were relatively inaccessible through the pelvis and major calyces, vascular arrest was undertaken in order to provide a dry operating field. To protect renal function during the period of ischaemia, the kidney was either cooled (hypothermia) or perfused with the purine nucleotide, inosine (which helps to prevent the development of acute tubular necrosis). At the end of the operation, a nephrostomy was left *in situ*, and any residual calculi shown on subsequent X-rays were dissolved by intrarenal perfusion of the kidney through the nephrostomy using hemiacidrin (renacidin).

This form of surgery has been superseded by percutaneous stone extraction. In this procedure, the first stage is the establishment of a nephrostomy tract, and stone disintegration is undertaken by using either ultrasound probes or electrohydraulic leads passed through the tract and placed in contact with the stone. As in the open operation, a nephrostomy tube is left in place and chemolysis can be undertaken as described above. The latest non-invasive technique for the removal of stones in the upper urinary tract is extracorporeal lithotripsy, which can be undertaken by the generation of either shock waves or ultrasound. In cases of surgery for infected stones, it is essential to provide adequate antibiotic cover, which must be continued until all the fragments of the stones are removed or voided. Any residual calculus material will inevitably lead to recurrent stone formation, and this probably accounts for the current 10% recurrence rate.

Patients with obstructed urinary tracts are more liable to this type of stone formation than those with a proteus infection and normal upper tracts. Furthermore, females are four times more likely to develop these infected stones than males; this may be due to their increased susceptibility to upper urinary tract infections, particularly when associated with pregnancy. These events lead to a distensible ureter and renal pelvis with relative urinary stagnation. Obstructive lesions must be removed or corrected, not only for the purposes of preserving renal function, but to ensure the prevention of recurrent stone formation. As in other forms of urinary calculus disease, it is essential that a large fluid intake is encouraged, not only to dilute the constituents responsible for stone formation, but also to ensure repeated and rapid turnover of urine in the collecting system. The increase in voiding of bacteria thus produced helps to prevent urinary tract infection becoming established. Acidification of the urine by taking large amounts of ascorbic acid (up to 1 g/day) is a useful adjunct to help discourage proteus or pseudomonas infection. The patient should be encouraged to test the urine with litmus paper to ensure that the therapy is proving successful.

It is not understood why only some patients with obstructed or distensible tracts and an infection due to a urea-splitting organism should develop calculi. Once again, urinary inhibitors have been invoked, but the evidence for these is inconclusive. The role played by urinary macromolecules is discussed later.

CALCIUM STONES

The majority of stones contain calcium, and the natural history of the recurrence rate for this group is 15% one year after the first stone episode, 45% after four years and 66% after nine years[3]. In only about 10% of calcium stone formers can an underlying disease be identified, and, of these, primary hyperparathyroidism is the most common. Other disorders, such as sarcoidosis, renal tubular acidosis and Cushing's syndrome, should be recognized and appropriate therapy instituted if stone recurrence is to be abolished. The recurrence rate of renal stones can be reduced to below 42% after five years[4] by the simple expedient of insisting on a high fluid intake (at least 3 L/day) and a moderate calcium diet (about 500 mg calcium per day). This has been described as 'the stone clinic effect', and must be taken into consideration when comparing the results of a drug-therapy group with a so-called non-treatment stone-forming group (since patients attending a stone clinic will inevitably be encouraged to undertake the simple measures described).

The six risk factors previously mentioned will now be considered.

(i) Volume

There is no doubt that by increasing the urine volume, stone formation is decreased, probably because the compounds which are involved in the formation of stones are diluted. There are other factors in the urine which interact with the crystalloids and enable calcium and oxalate to remain in solution, despite having exceeded the solubility product. In other words, a given amount of calcium and oxalate, which would crystallize when placed in a solution of water at a given pH and temperature, are held in solution when placed in urine, i.e. supersaturation is present. When further amounts of calcium and oxalate are added to the urine, spontaneous nucleation of crystals will occur; this is known as the formation product.

The area of supersaturation between the solubility product and the formation product is called the metastable zone. This phenomenon may well be due to the presence of organic molecules in the urine, variously known as urinary macromolecules (predominantly mucoproteins and mucopolysaccharides) or urinary colloids. These substances have a negative electrical charge, so that positively charged ions (such as calcium) are adsorbed on to their surfaces and consequently are taken out of solution. Such substances have been called crystallization inhibitors, a term which also encompasses citrates, pyrophosphates, and chondroitin sulphate, amongst others, resulting in some confusion and disagreement as to the roles played by these compounds in the evolution and inhibition of urolithiasis.

(ii) Urinary pH

Urinary pH determines the phosphate content of calcium phosphate stones, since the saturation or solubility product of calcium phosphate is more readily exceeded at a high pH. Phosphates in the diet (potatoes, bread, etc.) are an important source of urinary phosphate, which, with creatinine, are the main urinary buffers concerned with balancing the hydrogen ions excreted in the urine, and so determining the pH of the urine. The urinary creatinine level is mainly a function of the size of the muscle mass of the patient, and is little influenced by protein intake. With the exception of infected stones (*vide supra*), urinary pH is not a major risk factor in idiopathic calcium stone disease.

(iii) Urinary calcium

The measurements of serum and urinary calcium concentrations are commonly the first investigations undertaken by most practitioners presented with a patient afflicted with urinary calculus disease. In my own series of 400 undoubted stone formers, a calcium metabolic screen was normal in 61.5%. The urinary collections were undertaken on a free diet while the patients led a normal active life, and not while they were in hospital where the diet is not that taken at home or at work, and where mobility and exercise are restricted. It is illogical to record the patient's calcium metabolic state in artificial and unphysiological conditions. Three collections were taken over a three-week period at the convenience of the patient.

Other investigators claim that there is a calcium metabolic abnormality in 70% of stone patients they studied[5]. The disparity between these studies relates to the urinary calcium measurements, since, in my series, there were only eight patients (3%) with hypercalcaemia, six of whom underwent partial parathyroidectomies; these figures do not differ markedly from other reports from large local populations, as opposed to reports from specialized referral centres.

The definition of hypercalciuria is an arbitrary one. If the upper limit of normal daily urine calcium excretion in the male is stated to be 200 mg (5 mmol) per day on a 400 mg calcium diet[5], the percentage of men with hypercalciuria will be larger than in my series when only

28% of 100 known stone formers on a 400 mg calcium diet had a urinary calcium in excess of 300 mg (7.5 mmol) per day (my definition of hypercalciuria). Although it is of considerable interest and value to study the physiology of intestinal absorption and handling by the kidney (in stone patients) of a sizeable oral loading dose (1 g) of calcium[6], it must be questioned whether this justifies subdividing the patients with hypercalciuria into numerous subgroups and recommending different types of therapy – particularly since the results obtained are not those which pertain when patients are on a normal or restricted calcium intake. Furthermore, there is no practical advantage in defining different types of hypercalciuria, as the results of treating all hypercalciurics with thiazides[7] are very similar.

In a series of 108 patients[4] with idiopathic calcium urolithiasis seen at the Mayo Clinic, and followed for a mean of five years, a high fluid intake and sensible limitation of the intake of dairy products halted new stone formation or stone growth in 58% (including some with hypercalciuria). This has been called 'the stone clinic effect'. The authors recommended that all idiopathic stone formers should be managed on this simple conservative regime, and be carefully followed up for evidence of continuing urolithiasis. The minority who continue to exhibit active urolithiasis will then require detailed investigation and demand appropriate therapy. This approach of a continuing follow-up programme makes a considerable impact on the workload of a department and implies a special interest in stone disease. The cost effectiveness has to be compared with undertaking routine (three blood samples and three 24-hour urine collections) investigations of calcium measurements in all stone patients and discharging those with normal values from follow-up – recognizing that a sizeable number will continue to form new stones or have continued stone growth. This latter approach may be acceptable in a busy department committed to providing a comprehensive urological service to a large local population.

A further option is to prescribe thiazides as preventive therapy; these drugs are effective in lowering the urinary calcium excretion which is probably the most important risk factor in calcium stone disease. However, in a double-blind control clinical trial of 62 patients[8] with recurrent idiopathic renal calculi (irrespective of urinary calcium excretion levels), two groups were prescribed either 7.5 mg bendrofluazide daily or a placebo. Both groups demonstrated a similar reduction in stone formation. Recent studies[9] have shown that thiazides reduce urinary calcium excretion for three months, but, at six and twelve months, the levels revert to the pretreatment values. The observed reduction in stone formation is thus presumably due to 'the stone clinic effect' and there are convincing reasons for adopting the Mayo Clinic protocol described above.

(iv) Urinary oxalates

Urinary oxalates, together with calcium, form about 70% of stones seen in the Western world. A small increase in the urinary content of oxalate is ten times more potent than calcium in causing the precipitation of calcium oxalate. It follows that high levels of urinary oxalate are of considerable relevance; in patients with idiopathic calcium stones, less than 5% have an increase in urinary oxalate excretion (about 40 mg/day). About 10% of the urinary oxalates are dietary in origin.

The commonest cause of hyperoxaluria is gastrointestinal malabsorption which paradoxically causes increased absorption of dietary oxalate. This appears to be related to disturbances in bile salt metabolism with associated abnormalities of fatty acid and calcium handling in the gut. Hyperoxaluria is also noted in those patients who have had a by-pass procedure for obesity, or who, as a result of intestinal disease, have had a resection or a by-pass of a segment of the small intestine. This enterically acquired hyperoxaluria is further exaggerated by a low calcium diet. Since dietary calcium is normally bound to oxalate in the gut, any decrease in calcium causes the concentration of oxalate, in the form of free oxalate anions, to increase; these anions are then absorbed by the colon and so pass into the urine. Hence, dietary oxalates must be reduced; foods rich in this compound include strawberries, spinach, celery, chocolate, etc. A high calcium diet with a decreased oxalate intake is necessary in these circumstances. As an alternative to giving calcium (as a binding agent), aluminium (in the form of antacids) may be prescribed. To correct the failure of bile salt absorption, cholestyramine is given, in addition to enforcing a low-fat diet if steatorrhoea is present.

The majority of the urinary oxalates are the result of glyoxalate metabolism. Rare inherited (autosomal recessive) disorders, due to deficiency of specific enzymes, can lead to increased amounts of urinary excretion of oxalic acid. Type I hyperoxaluria is the commonest; there is an increased excretion of glycolic and oxalic acids. In Type II hyperoxaluria, the increase in oxalic acid excretion is accompanied by L-glyceric acids. Pyridoxine, (40 mg/day) in divided doses, is known to reduce oxalates in a proportion of these patients and should be given a trial.

(v) Uric acid

Uric acid is often a constituent of calcium stones, but the interrelationship between calcium and uric acid metabolism is poorly understood. Only a small number of idiopathic calcium stone formers have an increased excretion of urinary uric acid. It does appear, however, that the concentration of urinary uric acid affects calcium stone formation as a result of its activity on the acid mucopolysaccharide inhibitors. Workers in Israel[10] demonstrated that uric acid supersaturation is the result of the presence and properties of the Tamm-Horsfall mucoprotein. The amount and composition of these macromolecules, however, were similar in urine from normal subjects and from patients with idiopathic uric acid lithiasis. The difference between the two groups may lie in the size of the polymers of these mucoproteins (see below).

Patients with recurrent calcium oxalate calculi with elevated serum uric acid levels were given either allopurinol or a placebo[11], for a minimum period of six months, and, in some cases, for up to five years; in addition, they all alkalinized their urine and took an adequate fluid intake. As mentioned previously, 'the stone clinic effect' was evident in this study, with a decrease in stone formation activity in the placebo group but a greater decrease in those taking allopurinol, 61% of whom formed no further stones. It has been suggested that, by preventing uric acid crystalluria, the epitactic stimulus for the formation of calcium oxalate is avoided.

(vi) Urinary macromolecules

The part played by the urinary macromolecules in stone formation is confused and ill understood. In the first place, it is as well to establish what is meant by some of the terms used.

Macromolecules are high-molecular weight compounds (alternatively known as mucosubstances), best defined as proteins firmly bound to a carbohydrate (the latter containing hexosamine and/or hexose, sialic acid and fucose). Mucoproteins and mucopolysaccharides are both mucosubstances; in the former, the protein component predominates, while the carbohydrate is the major moiety in a mucopolysaccharide.

The most abundant mucoprotein found in urine is the Tamm–Horsfall mucoprotein, also called uromucoid. There are numerous polymers of Tamm–Horsfall mucoprotein, the largest being of 28 million daltons, and the lesser polymers measuring 14, 7, 3.5, and 1.7 million daltons. Immunologically, these are all identical and represent a number of polymers made up of repeating units arranged end-to-end and also side-to-side, linked by sialic acid molecules. Two-thirds of the urinary macromolecules in urine from normal individuals are smaller than 30 000 daltons, whereas, in stone formers, all macromolecules are larger than 50 000 daltons. If it is accepted that the negatively charged mucoprotein adsorbs calcium and other cations on to its surface, then the greater the subdivision of these mucosubstances, the greater the surface area available for this activity. Such adsorption thus chelates or takes calcium out of solution, and explains the presence of the metastable zone seen in normal urine – the solubility products of calcium and oxalate are exceeded, yet nucleation and crystallization are absent.

As the larger mucosubstances present in urine from stone formers have a decreased total surface area, a lesser amount of calcium is adsorbed on to these surfaces; hence, supersaturation and precipitation of crystalloids will occur. The factors which determine the size of the mucosubstances are unknown, but it is the author's opinion that the urinary proteolytic enzyme, plasmin (of fibrinolysis) is responsible. Further work is in progress in an attempt to resolve this question.

There are many mucopolysaccharides in urine, including hyaluronic acid, hexuronic acid, chondroitin sulphate, etc. The acidic mucopolysaccharides are now called glycosaminoglycans and they are said to inhibit the crystallization of urinary calcium salts.

There is another school of thought which states that the mucosubstances are an essential ingredient in the genesis of stone formation and form the skeletal framework on which the crystalloids adhere. It is not inconceivable that there should exist a dynamic equilibrium represented by a balance between the physical properties of colloidal (mucosubstances) dispersions, in which the particles tend to aggregate (van der Waals attractive forces) countered by the proteolytic enzymic activity of urinary fibrinolysis, the function of which is to depolymerize the urinary macromolecules. It seems likely that this is the most fruitful avenue to follow if stone recurrence is to be further decreased.

RECURRENCE AND CAUSES OF UROLITHIASIS

A further reduction in the recurrence of urinary calculi may be achieved by examining some of the factors which may have been responsible for converting a non-stone forming race or culture into a stone-forming population.

Renal stone disease is virtually unknown in the Bantu living in South Africa[13], yet, when members of the race are translocated to America, their successors (the American negro) form renal stones as commonly as the rest of the American population[14]. It is not possible for a genetic change to occur in a cohort within a few generations, and so any changes must be attributable to an altered environment or diet. It should be noted that coronary thrombosis is similarly rare in the Bantu in Africa, but, after becoming Westernized, the prevalence rises markedly, approaching that of the indigenous population[15].

These observations are supported by work undertaken 47 years ago, when 1060 kidneys were dissected by Vermooten in South Africa[13]. Four years previously, Randall[16] had described calcified plaques on the renal papilla, which, in his view, provided the nidus of renal calculi. Vermooten found that Randall's plaques were present in 4.3% of the Bantus but in 17.2% of those of Caucasian stock; he also observed a relative increase in these plaques in patients with cardiovascular disease – especially in the 50–70 age group. These findings led him to speculate as to whether there was a connection between the disease processes responsible for arteriosclerosis and the deposition of Randall's plaque.

Comparisons of protein intake and fat consumption with hospital incidence of urolithiasis, as observed in three areas with differing levels of economic development[17], demonstrate that there is a direct correlation between stone incidence and the dietary intake of protein and fat, not dissimilar to that seen in cardiovascular degenerative disease.

Recently, Professor Blacklock's urological unit in Manchester has pursued (personal communication) the association of urolithiasis and arteriosclerosis in terms of nutrients, diet and risk factors, and noted that the plasma cholesterol and triglyceride concentrations were higher in nine male stone formers than in eleven normal subjects. Prospective epidemiological studies are required to determine if there is any relationship between arterial and cardiovascular disease, on the one hand, and the prevalence of stone disease on the other, bearing in mind that the dietary risk factors for urolithiasis and degenerative arterial disease are similar.

References

1. Marickar, Y. M. F. and Rose, G. A. (1985). Relation of stone growth and urinary biochemistry in long-term follow-up of stone patients with idiopathic hypercalciuria. *Br. J. Urol.*, **57**, 613–17
2. Robertson, W. G., Peacock, M., Heyburn, P. J., Marshall, D. H. and Clark, P. J. (1978). Risk factors in calcium stone disease of the urinary tract. *Br. J. Urol.*, **50**, 449–54
3. Coe, F. L. (1980). Clinical stone disease. In Coe, F. L., Brenner, S. M. and Stein, J. H. (eds.) *Nephrolithiasis, Contemporary Issues in Nephrology*, pp. 1–12. (New York: Churchill Livingstone)
4. Hosking, D. H., Erickson, S. B., Van den Berg, C. J., Wilson, D. M. and Smith, L. H. (1983). The stone clinic effect in patients with idiopathic calcium urolithiasis. *J. Urol.*, **130**, 1115–18
5. Pak, C. Y. C., Britton, F., Peterson, R., Ward, D., Northcutt, C., Breslau, N. A., McGuire, J., Sakhaee, K., Bush, S., Nicar, M., Norman, D. A. and Peters, P. (1980). Ambulatory evaluation of nephrolithiasis. Classification, clinical presentation and diagnostic criteria. *Am. J. Med.*, **69**, 19–30
6. Pak, C. Y. C. (1982). Medical management of nephrolithiasis. *J. Urol.*, **128**, 1157–64
7. Elomaa, I., Ala-Opas, M. and Porkaa, L. (1984). Five years of experience with selective therapy in recurrent calcium nephrolithiasis. *J. Urol.*, **132**, 656–61
8. Brocks, P., Dahl, C. and Wolf, H. (1981). Do thiazides prevent idiopathic renal calcium stones? *Lancet*, **2**, 124–5

9. Kohri, K., Takada, M., Katoh, Y., Kataoka, K., Ihuchi, M., Yachiku, S. and Kurita, T. (1987). Parathyroid hormone and electrolytes during long-term treatment with allopurinol and thiazide. *Br. J. Urol.*, **59,** 503–7
10. Sperling, O., de Vries, A. and Kedem, O. (1965). Studies on the etiology of uric acid lithiasis. IV. Urinary non-dialysable substances in idiopathic uric acid lithiasis. *J. Urol.*, **94,** 286–92.
11. Smith, M. J. V. (1977). Placebo versus allopurinol for renal calculi. *J. Urol.*, **117,** 690–2
12. Drach, G. W., Kraljevich, Z. and Randolph, A. D. (1982). Effects of high molecular weight urinary macromolecules on crystallization of calcium oxalate dihydrate. *J. Urol.*, **127,** 805–10
13. Vermooten, V. (1941). The incidence and significance of the deposition of calcium plaques in the renal papilla as observed in the caucasian and negro (Bantu) population in South Africa. *J. Urol.*, **46,** 193–200
14. Dodson, A. I. and Clark, J. R. (1946). Incidence of urinary calculi in the American negro. *J. Am. Med. Assoc.*, **132,** 1063–6
15. Meade, T. W., Brozovic, M., Chakrabarti, R., Haines, A. P., North, W. R. S. and Stirling, Y. (1978). Ethnic group comparisons of variables associated with ischaemic heart disease. *Br. Heart J.*, **40,** 789–95.
16. Randall, A. (1937). The origin and growth of renal calculi. *Ann. Surg.*, **105,** 1009–27
17. Anderson, D. A. (1973). Environmental factors in the aetiology of urolithiasis. In Cifuentes Delatte, L., Rapado, A. and Hodgkinson, A. (eds.) *Urinary Calculi: Proceedings of International Symposium of Renal Stone Research*, pp. 130–44 (Basle: Karger)

4
CYSTINURIA

R. S. C. RODGER

INTRODUCTION

Defective transport of the amino acids, cystine, lysine, ornithine and arginine, in the renal proximal tubular cell resulting in aminoaciduria is the hallmark of cystinuria. Transport systems in the small intestine are also affected, leading to malabsorption of these amino acids (Figure 4.1). The biochemical defects will be referred to but have been reviewed extensively elsewhere[1-3]. The disorder, which is inherited in an autosomal recessive pattern, is called cystinuria because the important clinical features are related to the formation of cystine stones in the renal tract. Cystine and arginine excretion are equivalent and less than lysine excretion[4]. There are no important clinical effects caused by excessive dibasic amino acid excretion but the low solubility of cystine leads to its ready crystallization and subsequent calculus formation.

Cystinuria was first described in 1810 in a lecture by Wollaston to the Royal Society of London[5]. He described bladder calculi which he believed to be composed of an oxide because they were soluble in strong acid and alkali. It was later recognized that the compound was not an oxide but the amino acid, cystine. Garrod, in 1908[6], was first to suggest that the condition might be an inborn error of metabolism but it was Dent and Rose's hypothesis, following their work in 1951, that cystinuria was an inborn error of transport[7].

The disorder has been recognized in other mammals since 1823 when cystine calculi were reported in a dog[8] and most recently in the

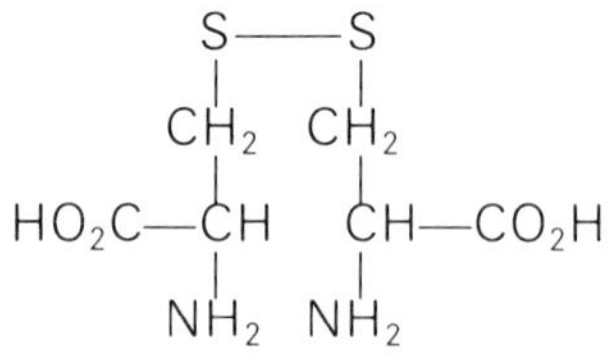

CALCULUS DISEASE

$$\begin{array}{cc} S\!\!-\!\!\!-\!\!S \\ | & | \\ CH_2 & CH_2 \\ | & | \\ HO_2C\!-\!CH & CH\!-\!CO_2H \\ | & | \\ NH_2 & NH_2 \end{array}$$

CYSTINE

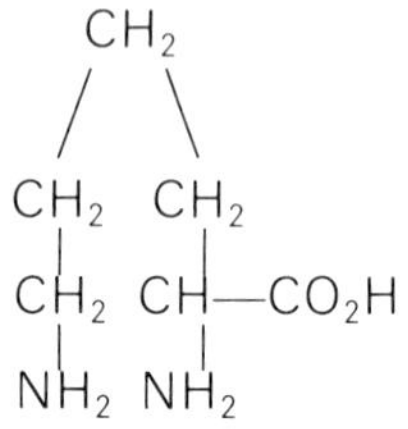

LYSINE

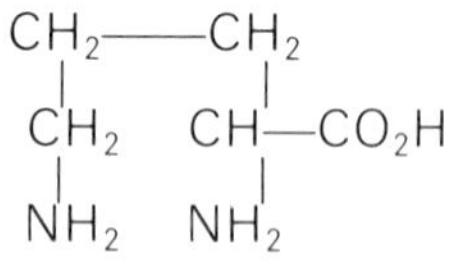

ORNITHINE

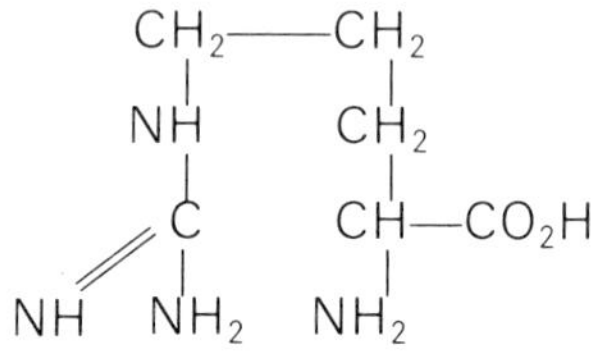

ARGININE

FIGURE 4.1 The amino acids whose transport is defective in cystinuria

Brazilian maned wolf[9]. Indeed, cystine stones accounted for 18% of renal calculi in a study of dogs in England[10] and were present in 10% of the wolves studied by Bovée et al.[11].

In the last twenty years, there have been considerable improvements in the treatment of cystinuria. Furthermore, renal replacement therapy is now readily available for those patients who develop progressive renal impairment. For these reasons, much of the clinical literature on cystinuria reported before 1970 is now unreliable. This review attempts to highlight the more recent studies concerning the clinical aspects of this condition.

CLINICAL FEATURES

Cystinuria accounts for 1–3% of all urinary stones and is a more frequent cause of calculi in children. Estimates of the prevalence of cystinuria in the general population vary considerably. In the United Kingdom, Crawhall and Watts, using Brand's screening test (see section on Diagnosis), examined urine samples from 1060 patients attending a medical out-patient department and found five with increased cystine concentration[12]. Further analysis of the urine of these subjects showed that their amino acid excretion profiles were indistinguishable from a group of heterozygotes. Using the assumption that the commonest type of cystinuria accounts for two thirds of all clinical cases, this study indicated that the prevalence of cystinuria was fifty per million population or 1/20 000. Results from a survey of 1000 university students in London provided a similar estimate[13]. Earlier surveys, where the disorder was found to be less common, probably failed to detect all heterozygotes. There appears to be considerable geographical variation in the incidence of cystinuria. In Sweden, ten persons per million population or 1/100 000 are said to be affected[14]. A joint study of neonatal screening demonstrated that the disorder was four times more frequent in Australia than America[15]. Although cystinuria occurs with equal frequency in both sexes, it had been suggested that males were more severely affected, and the explanation for this was that they had a greater likelihood of developing urethral calculus obstruction. Recent studies do not confirm this suggestion; in fact, in Smith and Wilcken's review of 110 cases, there was a preponderance of females with calculus disease[16].

Patients with cystinuria present with symptoms of urolithiasis or secondary complications, such as infection, hypertension and renal failure. Most present in the second and third decades although symptoms may occur at any age. For example, in one series[16], 7% of patients aged 5–15 years had calculi compared with 62% of patients aged 20–25. Long-term follow-up of homozygous cystinurics indicates that most will develop urinary calculus disease, although this may be reduced with the current improvements in therapy which are available.

Urinary tract infections may occur in up to one third of patients with cystinuria and are much more common in females[17]. Suspected infection should be proven by urine microscopy and culture, since crystalluria may also result in loin pain, dysuria and frequency. The incidence of hypertension increases with progressive renal impairment and is present in approximately 10% of patients in recent reviews[16,17].

There is some controversy about whether cystinurics have impaired growth: this might arise because of failure to absorb amino acids with consequent low plasma levels, and would be more likely in patients with repeated infections or renal impairment. Furthermore, there is some evidence that cystinurics have abnormal zinc metabolism[18], and zinc deficiency is known to cause impaired growth and sexual development in adolescents[19]. Several studies have shown that cystinurics have a lower mean height than age and sex matched controls, although a recent American study found no such difference[16,17,20]. In their review of 110 cystinurics in Australia, Smith and Wilcken showed that both males and females were 4 cm shorter than figures reported for normal eighteen-year-old controls[16]. Furthermore, they found that unaffected siblings were significantly taller than homozygous cystinurics.

A neurological defect has been postulated based on three case reports of cystinuric patients developing central nervous system lesions with spastic paraplegia[21–23]. Blackburn and McLeod suggested that this was more than a chance association and speculated that an amino acid transport defect existed within the nervous system[23]. There is no direct evidence to support this although Scriver *et al.* and Wadman and Van Sprang, in separate studies, found a ten-fold increase in the incidence of cystinuria in mentally retarded populations[24,25]. Although there may be an association between cystinuria and mental retardation, the study of Gold *et al.* strongly suggested that it is only an association and not a direct effect of the metabolic disturbance[26].

He found no difference in intelligence testing between patients with cystinuria and unaffected siblings or controls.

The other main controversy about disorders associated with cystinuria concerns hyperuricaemia and gout. Melani and Canary described hyperuricaemia in four out of six cystinuric patients[27], and Vergis and Walker reported a patient with cystinuria who passed pure uric acid stones[28]. More recent reports provide further evidence of an association between cystinuria and gout. 30% of the patients in the Mayo series had hyperuricaemia and 23% of the male cystinurics in Smith and Wilcken's study had clinical gout compared with less than 2% of men in the general population[16,17].

Recent evidence also suggests that cystinurics have near normal fertility where renal function is conserved. Gregory and Mansell[29] reported 41 normal births in 46 pregnancies in female cystinurics on conventional treatment. Although new stones developed in eighteen pregnancies, none required removal. Hypertension and urinary tract infection occurred in six pregnancies and all patients continued to have normal renal function. There is no contraindication to breast feeding in such patients as amino acid profiles of breast milk are normal[30]. This latter point indicates that the amino acid transport defect in cystinuria does not affect the breast duct epithelium.

With improvements in the therapy of cystinuria and in the management of chronic renal failure in general, it is hoped that cystinurics should have a near normal life expectancy. Prior to 1960, the average longevity of men with cystinuria was 37 years[31]. A Swedish series later gave an average life expectancy of 52 years for men and 64 years for women[14]. Current series show no sex difference in survival and a much lower incidence of renal failure which was previously the main cause of death[17].

DIAGNOSIS

Routine urinalysis is abnormal in most patients with cystinuria, 90% showing mild proteinuria or microscopic haematuria. Hexagonal crystals, which are pathognomonic, may be seen on light-microscopic examination of a concentrated urine sample. The normal cystine excretion is 40–80 mg/day but 80% of homozygous cystinurics excrete in excess of 500 mg/day. A screening test (the Brand's test) is available, based on the addition of 5% sodium cyanide, and later sodium nitroprusside, to a sample of urine. A positive test is indicated by the presence of a magenta colour. The test may be positive in other conditions such as acetonuria and homocystinuria. A modified kit test has recently been described[32] using Ames ketosticks, which has a sensitivity for cystine of 50 mg/L.

Plasma cystine levels are not measured routinely but, along with the dibasic amino acids, are on average slightly low. Urinary excretion of putrescine and cadaverine, the breakdown products of lysine and arginine released by intestinal bacteria, are also increased.

Cystine stones usually have a smooth and waxy yellowish appearance. In 50–70% of cases, they consist of pure cystine, whilst the majority of the remainder contain small amounts of hydroxyapatite and ammonium magnesium phosphate[14]. Other stone compositions, including non-cystine stones, have been described but are rare[33].

The stones may be small or may form staghorn calculi. In 25% of cases, they are said to be bilateral and they are usually found in sterile urine. The sulphur content of cystine renders them less radio-opaque than calcium stones and small ureteric calculi may be overlooked.

MANAGEMENT

Supersaturation of the urine with cystine leads to the precipitation of hexagonal crystals which coalesce to form small calculi. The solubility of cystine is pH dependent and is also influenced by the electrolyte and macromolecule content of the urine[34]; however specific inhibitors of crystal formation have not been recognized. The principles of treatment are to reduce the urinary excretion and concentration of cystine and to increase its solubility by optimizing the urinary pH. This can be effective in preventing the formation and promoting the dissolution of calculi.

Diet

Dietary restriction of protein, or specifically of methionine, the essential amino acid which is the precursor of cystine, reduces cystine excretion but is poorly tolerated. Furthermore, protein restriction may lead to malnutrition in patients with severe cystinuria. Equivalent doses of vegetable protein are associated with much lower levels of cystine excretion than animal protein and so patients should be advised to avoid a high-protein intake and to moderate their consumption of animal protein[35].

An exciting development has been the discovery that amino acid excretion can be reduced by dietary sodium restriction. Jaeger *et al.*[36] studied four patients with cystinuria, examining the effects of glutamine on cystine excretion (see below). They found that glutamine was effective in reducing cystine excretion in patients with high, but not low, sodium intakes. They went on to demonstrate that sodium restriction alone, from 300 to 150 mmol/day, reduced amino acid excretion by half. If these results are confirmed, dietary sodium restriction could be an important addition to the therapy of cystinuria and might replace alkalinization of the urine because of the high sodium load that this involves.

Fluid

The solubility of cystine in the pH range 4.5–7.5 is 250–300 mg/L. Since most cystinurics excrete more than 500 mg cystine per day, crystalluria and stone formation are likely to occur with urine flows below 150 ml/h. In addition to pH changes, the presence of electrolytes and macromolecules in the urine alters the solubility profile of cystine. This may explain, in part, the variable susceptibility of cystinurics to stone formation. High fluid regimes should be encouraged as they have been shown, not only to prevent calculus disease, but also to promote stone dissolution[37]. Patients should be advised to maintain an even intake of fluid throughout the 24 h period as stone formation is said to occur in many patients overnight. The institution and maintenance of satisfactory high fluid regimes requires careful explanation to obtain maximal co-operation and this may be particularly difficult in children[38].

Alkali

Alkalinization of the urine increases the solubility of cystine. However, to be effective, a urinary pH of 7.5–8 must be maintained. This is difficult to achieve with oral therapy, requiring 10–30 g sodium bicarbonate daily, but will double the solubility of cystine in the urine. Acetazolamide may be used to facilitate alkalinization but may itself cause crystalluria if the patient does not adhere to a high fluid regime. Alkalinization of the urine may result in sodium retention and heart failure in elderly patients and a metabolic alkalosis in children. In addition, it will predispose to nephrocalcinosis and calcium-containing calculi by rendering the urine less soluble to calcium and phosphate[39].

Sulphadryl therapy

Cystine is a disulphide neutral amino acid and, as such, will react with other sulphides to form mixed disulphides (Figure 4.2). These mixed disulphides are much more soluble than cystine and this is the rationale for therapy with sulphadryl compounds, such as penicillamine and mercaptopropionylglycine.

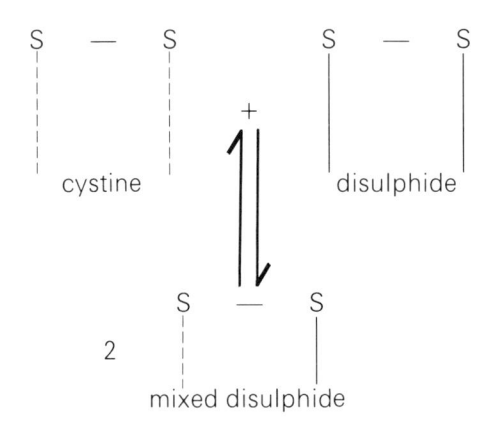

FIGURE 4.2   The disulphide reaction

Penicillamine

Successful treatment with this drug in cystinurics was first reported by Crawhall *et al.* in 1963[40]. It is effective in reducing cystine excretion below 200 mg/L, thus preventing stone formation and allowing dissolution of existing calculi[41]. The drug is given three or four times daily to a total dose of 1–2 g but has major problems with patient acceptability and toxicity. It is unpleasant to take and is frequently associated with nausea, vomiting and abdominal pain. Sensitivity reactions, manifested by skin rash, fever, arthralgia and lymphadenopathy, occur in the first two weeks of therapy in up to 50% of patients[42]. The drug may be successfully reintroduced with steroid cover or after a period of desensitization. Altered taste acuity may occur with penicillamine treatment and is said to be prevented by prophylactic pyridoxine treatment[43]. It may also be a feature of trace metal deficiency and is said to be improved by replacement with copper[44]. Renal, haematological and autoimmune side effects are most serious. Penicillamine is well recognized as causing membranous nephropathy and the nephrotic syndrome[45] but other forms of nephritis, including rapidly progressive glomerulonephritis, have been described[46]. The haematological manifestations of toxicity are leucopenia and thrombocytopenia but occasionally thrombocytosis may occur[47]. Autoimmune disturbances include the development of autoantibodies, lupus erythematosus and myasthenia gravis[48,49].

Approximately 50% of patients are unable to tolerate penicillamine because of its side effects. The drug should be introduced at a low dose which should be increased gradually. Patients should be seen frequently initially and their haematological and biochemical indices and urinary protein excretion should continue to be monitored in the longer term, as complications may develop late in treatment. Because of its toxicity, penicillamine is generally not used prophylactically in patients with cystinuria, but is reserved for patients with troublesome calculus disease uncontrolled by conservative treatment.

Mercaptopropionylglycine (MPG)

This agent has been studied in an attempt to find a less toxic agent than penicillamine. It was shown to be one and a half times as effective as penicillamine in reducing cystine excretion on a weight-for-weight basis in both long- and short-term studies in small numbers of patients[50]. Although there is less long-term experience with MPG, a large study from Texas reported in 1986 and supported the view that it is a useful alternative to penicillamine[51]. It produced remission of stone formation in over 60% of patients and reduced the individual stone formation rate in over 80% of patients. A high incidence of side effects was reported, however, and 30% of patients had reactions necessitating withdrawal of treatment. Toxicity was less than with penicillamine, but one of the criteria for entry to the study was penicillamine intolerance. The side-effect profile with MPG is similar to that of penicillamine and further experience is needed to determine whether it is less toxic.

Captoril

The first report of this antihypertensive agent, which contains a sulphadryl group, being used in the treatment of cystinuria has only recently been published[52]. This preliminary study in two patients noted that it was effective and well tolerated over 2–3 months of treatment.

Glutamine

There have been conflicting reports on the effect of this agent on urinary cystine excretion. In 1979, Miyagi *et al.* demonstrated a significant reduction in cystine excretion in one patient[53]. This work was not confirmed in subsequent studies until the recent report of Jaegar *et al.*[36] whose observations led to the conclusion that the anticystinuric effects of glutamine are dependent on sodium intake. Unlike the sulphadryl compounds, glutamine is well tolerated and safe to use. It therefore may prove to have a place in the treatment of cystinuria in patients unable to comply with sodium restriction.

Other medical treatment

Other medical measures proposed include the administration of choline, naphthaline and vitamin A. These agents are generally held to be ineffective. A report in 1983 by Lux and May, however, recorded a 70% reduction in cystine following 3–5 g oral ascorbic acid therapy[54]. Follow-up intravenous urography showed that none of the four patients had recurrence of cystine stone formation. Ascorbic acid is well tolerated and its action is to promote the reduction of cystine to cysteine. It does, however, have the potential for increasing oxalate excretion, particularly in patients with impaired renal function[55].

Surgery

Despite the improvements in medical treatment, many patients still require surgery for the relief of obstruction or removal of large stones after medical treatment of cystinuria has been instituted. Surgery may be more often required when stones are associated with infection. Cystine stones are amenable to the newer methods of removal, including extracorporeal shock wave lithotripsy, although they are more resistant to this latest treatment than stones of other chemical composition[56].

Renal replacement therapy

Although the proportion of cystinurics who develop renal impairment is falling, a number will continue to require renal replacement therapy. The progression of renal failure should be treated along standard conservative lines with control of hypertension and phosphate and the prompt eradication of infection. Moderate protein restriction may also be helpful as long as care is taken to ensure that the patient does not develop malnutrition. Cystinurics who develop end-stage renal failure should have a good prognosis on renal replacement therapy as they are often young and do not have a systemic disease. Patients may be maintained on haemodialysis or peritoneal dialysis (CAPD) and considered for renal transplantation. A number of reports have demonstrated that, as expected, the urinary amino acid excretion returns to normal post-transplantation[57,58].

GENETIC COUNSELLING

The gene for the cystinuria transport system has yet to be cloned and mapped to a specific chromosome locus. Cystinuria is considered an autosomal recessive condition, since all patients who develop stones are homozygotes. By measuring urinary amino acid excretion in family members, Harris and Warren differentiated the completely recessive type, who had normal amino acid excretion, from the incompletely recessive variant where the excretion of cystine and lysine are increased[59].

Rosenberg *et al.*[60] classified cystinuria according to the response of plasma cystine to an oral cystine load and amino acid transport of the small intestine *in vitro*. He defined three heterozygote types: type I corresponding to recessive cystinuria with normal amino acid excretion in heterozygotes, no transport defect of amino acids in the small intestine and no change in plasma cystine following an oral load. Types II and III comprised the incompletely recessive cystinurics. In type II, the urinary excretion of cystine and lysine are increased, there is slight reduction in cystine transport in the small intestine and a slight rise in plasma cystine levels following an oral load. In type III, cystine and lysine excretion in the urine are increased, the intestinal transport of cystine and lysine are impaired and there is a subnormal rise in plasma cystine following an oral load. In spite of the heterogenicity of heterozygous individuals, there are no clinical features to differentiate types I, II and III homozygotes.

In clinical practice, it is important to distinguish homozygotes from heterozygotes and normals. Urinary screening tests will detect homozygotes, a proportion of heterozygotes and will include a few false positive patients, such as those with acetonuria. Homozygotes will be clearly recognized by quantitative measurement of their urinary amino acid excretion, except in early infancy. Heterozygous infants under six months of age can excrete amino acids in the range found in homozygous adults[61].

Although heterozygotes for cystinuria do not develop cystine stones, they may have an increased incidence of calcium oxalate calculi. Resnick et al.[62] found that 13.4% of recurrent calcium oxalate stone formers were heterozygotes for cystinuria, although this was not confirmed in a later study in a different region[63].

ISOLATED CYSTINURIA

Increased urinary excretion of cystine with normal dibasic amino acid excretion has been reported in two children[64]. This is believed to be due to a specific transport defect in the brush border membrane of the renal tubule for the reabsorption of cystine. There have also been reports from family studies of patients with isolated dibasic aminoaciduria and isolated lysinuria. These aminoacidurias are also due to defects of specific amino acid transport systems in the renal tubule but are not of importance clinically.

SUMMARY

Cystinuria is a rare autosomal recessive disorder which, in homozygotes, frequently leads to the development of calculus disease in early adult life. The disorder is caused by a defect in the transport system for cystine and dibasic amino acids in the proximal renal tubule and small intestine. The clinical features are those of crystalluria, urolithiasis and its secondary complications. The standard treatment is to avoid a high intake of animal protein and to maintain a high fluid intake. Resistant cases may be treated by sulphadryl compounds but these carry a high likelihood of toxicity. The role of other therapeutic regimes, such as alkalinization, sodium restriction, glutamine and ascorbic acid, is currently in flux.

Acknowledgements

I am grateful to Miss Anne T. McFadden who prepared the manuscript.

References

1. Watts, R. W. E. (1976). Cystinuria. In Chisholm, G. D. and Innes Williams, D. *Urology*, 1st Edn. (London: Heinemann)
2. Scriver, C. R. (1986). Cystinuria. *N. Engl. J. Med.*, **315,** 1155
3. Thiers, S. O. and Halperin, E. C. (1980). Cystinuria. In Coe, F. L. (Ed.) *Nephrolithiasis*. (New York: Churchill Livingstone)
4. Crawhall, J. C., Purkiss, P., Watts, R. W. E. and Young, E. P. (1969). The excretion of amino acids by cystinuria patients and their relatives. *Ann. Hum. Genet.*, **33,** 149
5. Wollaston, W. H. (1810). On cystic oxide a new species of urinary calculus. *Trans. R. Soc. London*, **100,** 223
6. Garrod, A. E. (1908). Inborn errors of metabolism. *Lancet*, **2,** 142 and 124
7. Dent, C. E. and Rose, G. A. (1951). Aminoacid metabolism in cystinuria. *Q. J. Med.*, **20,** 205
8. Lassaigne, J. L. (1823). Observation sur l'existence de l'oxide cystique dans un calcul vesical du chien. *Ann. Chim. Phys.*, 2nd Ser, **23,** 328
9. Bush, M. and Bovee, K. C. (1978) Cystinuria in the maned wolf. *J. Am. Vet. Med. Assoc.*, **173,** 1159
10. White, E. G. T., Treacher, R. J. and Porter, P. (1961). Urinary calculi in the dog. Incidence and chemical composition. *J. Comp. Pathol.*, **71,** 201
11. Bovée, K. C., Bush, M., Dietz, J., Jezyk, P. and Segal, S. (1981). Cystinuria in the maned wolf of South America. *Science*, **212,** 919
12. Crawhall, J. C. and Watts, R. W. E. (1968). Cystinuria. *Am. J. Med.*, **45,** 746
13. Mallison, Quoted by Harris, H. and Warren, F. G. (1953). Quantitative studies on the urinary cystine in patients with cystine stone formation and their relations. *Ann. Eugen.*, **18,** 125
14. Bostrom, H. and Hambraeus, L. (1964). Cystinuria in Sweden. VII. Clinical histopathological and medico social aspects of the disease. *Acta Med. Scand.*, S **411**
15. Levy, H. (1973). Genetic screening. In Herns, H. and Hirschorn, K. (eds.) *Advances in Human Genetics*, Vol. 4, p. 1. (New York: Plenum Press)
16. Smith, A. and Wilcken, B. (1984). Homozygous cystinuria in New South Wales. *Med. J. Aust.*, **141,** 500
17. Dahlberg, P. J., Van Den Berg, C. J., Kurtz, S. B., Wison, D. W. and Smith, L. H. (1977). Clinical features and management of cystinuria. *Mayo Clin. Proc.*, **52,** 533
18. Ruse, W., Keeling, P. W. N., Thompson, R. P. H. and Maxwell, M. A. (1982). Zinc and cystinuria. *Clin. Sci.*, **63,** 223
19. Prader, A. S., Schulert, A. R., Miale, A., Farid, Z. and Sanstead, H. H. (1963). Zinc and iron deficiency in male subjects with dwarfism and hypogonadism but without acyclostomiasis. *Am. J. Clin. Nutr.*, **12,** 437
20. Collis, J. E., Levi, A. J. and Milne, M. D. (1963). Structure and nutrition in cystinuria and Hartnup disease. *Br. Med. J.*, **1,** 590
21. Banerji, N. K. and Millar, J. H. E. (1971). Paraplegia associated with cystinuria. *J. Neurol. Sci.*, **12,** 101
22. De Myer, W. and Gebbard, R. L. (1975). Subacute combined degeneration of the spinal cord with cystinuria. *Neurology*, **25,** 994

23. Blackburn, C. R. B. and McLeod, J. G. (1977). CNS lesions in cystinuria. *Arch. Neurol.*, **34,** 638
24. Scriver, C. R., Whelon, D. T., Clow, C. L. and Dallaire, L. (1970). Cystinuria: Increased prevalence in patients with mental disease. *N. Engl. J. Med.*, **283,** 783
25. Wadman, S. K. and Van Sprang, F. J. (1971). Frequency of mental retardation and neurological disturbances in patients with cystinuria. In Carson, N. A. J. and Raine, D. M. (eds.) *Inherited Disorders of Sulfur Metabolism*, p. 81. (London; Churchill Livingstone)
26. Gold, R. J. M., Dobrinski, M. J. and Gold, D. P. (1977). Cystinuria and mental deficiency. *Clin. Gen.*, **12,** 329
27. Melani, C. R. and Canary, J. J. (1967). Cystinuria with hyperuricemia. *J. Am. Med. Assoc.*, **200,** 169
28. Vergis, J. G. and Walker, B. R. (1970). Cystinuria, hyperuricaemia and uric acid nephrolithiasis. *Nephron*, **7,** 577
29. Gregory, M. C. and Mansell, M. A. (1983). Pregnancy and cystinuria. *Lancet*, **2,** 1158
30. Gahl, W. A. and Rizzo, W. B. (1983). Normal free dibasic amino acids in breast milk of a woman with cystinuria. *N. Engl. J. Med.*, **309,** 1388
31. Renander, A. (1941). The roentgen density of the cystine calculus. *Acta Radiol.*, **S41**
32. David, R. M., Shihabi, Z. K. and O'Connor, M. L. (1986). Simplified method for cystinuria screening. *Clin. Chem.*, **32,** 1417
33. Evans, W. P., Resnick, M. I. and Bozce, W. H. (1982). Homozygous cystinuria – evaluation of 35 patients. *J. Urol.*, **127,** 707
34. Pak, C. Y. C. and Fuller, C. Y. J. (1983). Assessment of cystine solubility in urine and of heterogenous nucleation. *J. Urol.*, **129,** 1066
35. Rodman, J. S., Blackburn, P., Williams, J. J., Brown, A., Pospischil, M. A. and Peterson, C. M. (1984). The effect of dietary protein on cystine excretion in a patient with cystinuria. *Clin. Nephrol.*, **22,** 273
36. Jaeger, P., Portman, L., Saunders, A., Rosenberg, L. E. and Thier, S. O. (1986). Anti cystinuric effects of glutamine and of dietary sodium restriction. *N. Engl. J. Med.*, **315,** 1120
37. Dent, C., Friedman, M., Green, H. and Watson, L. (1965). Treatment of cystinuria. *Br. Med. J.*, **1,** 403
38. MacDonald, W. B. and Selvarajah, K. (1976). The longterm management of cystinuria. *Aust. Paed. J.*, **12,** 102
39. Rosenburg, L. E. and Scriver, C. R. (1974). Cystinuria. In Duncan's *Diseases of Metabolism: Genetics and Metabolism*, p. 502. (Philadelphia: Saunders)
40. Crawhall, J. C., Scowen, E. F. and Watts, R. (1963). Effect of penicillamine on cystinuria. *Br. Med. J.*, **1,** 588
41. McDonald, J. E. and Henneman, P. H. (1965). Stone dissolution in vivo and control of cystinuria with D-penicillamine. *N. Engl. J. Med.*, **273,** 578
42. Stephens, A. D. and Watts, R. W. E. (1971). The treatment of cystinuria in *N*-acetyl-D-penicillamine, a comparison with the results of D-penicillamine treatment. *Q. J. Med.*, **40,** 355
43. Gibbs, K. and Walshe, J. M. (1966). Penicillamine and pyridoxine requirements in men. *Lancet*, **1,** 175
44. Bostrom, H. and Wester, P. O. (1967). Excretion of trace elements in two penicillamine treated cases of cystinuria. *Acta Med. Scand.*, **181,** 475

45. Jaffe, I. A., Treser, G., Suzuki, Y. and Ehrenreich, T. (1968). Nephropathy induced by D-penicillamine. *Ann. Int. Med.*, **69,** 549
46. Strenlieb, I., Bennet, B. and Scheinber, J. I. H. (1975). D-Penicillamine induced Goodpasture's syndrome in Wilson's disease. *Ann. Int. Med.*, **82,** 673
47. Ahmed, F., Sumalnap, V., Spain, D. M. and Jobin, M. S. (1978). Thrombohemolytic thrombocytopenic purpura during penicillamine therapy. *Arch. Int. Med.*, **138,** 1292
48. Appelboom, T., de Maubeuge, J., Unger, J. and Famaey, J. P. (1978). Cutaneous lupus induced by penicillamine. *Scand. J. Rheumatol.*, **7,** 64
49. Argov, L. and Mastalgia, F. L. (1979). Disorders of neuromuscular transmission caused by drugs. *N. Engl. J. Med.*, **301,** 409
50. Harber, J. A., Cusworth, D. C., Lauves, L. C. and Wrong, O. M. (1986). Comparison of 2 mercaptopropionglycine and D-penicillamine in the treatment of cystinuria. *J. Urol.*, **136,** 146
51. Pak, C. Y. C., Fuller, C., Sakhaee, K., Zerwekh, J. E. and Adams, B. V. (1986). Management of cystine nephrolithiasis with alpha mercaptopropionylglycine. *J. Urol.*, **136,** 1003
52. Gloand, J. A. and Izzo, J. L. (1987). Captopril reduces urinary cystine excretion in cystinurics. *Arch. Intern. Med.*, **147,** 1409
53. Miyagi, K., Nakada, F. and Ohshiro, S. (1979). Effect of glutamine on cystine excretion in a patient with cystinuria. *N. Engl. J. Med.*, **301,** 196
54. Lux, B. and May, P. (1983). Longterm observation of young cystinuric patients under ascorbic acid therapy. *Urol. Int.*, **38,** 91
55. Ono, K. (1986). Secondary hyperoxalemia caused by vitamin C supplementation in regular hemodialysis patients. *Clin. Nephrol.*, **26,** 239
56. Lingeman, J. E., Newman, D., Mertz, J. H. O., Mosbaugh, P. G., Steel, R. E., Kahoski, R. J., Cowry, T. A. and Woods, J. R. (1986). Extracorporeal short wave lithotrypsy: the Methodist Hospital of Indiana experience. *J. Urol.*, **135,** 1134
57. Kelly, S. and Nolan, G. P. (1983). Excretory rates in a post-transplant cystinuric patient. *J. Am. Med. Assoc.*, **239,** 1132
58. Hoitsma, A. J., Kocne, R. A. P., Trizbels, F. J. M. and Monmens, L. A. H. (1983). Disappearance of cystinuria after renal transplantation. *J. Am. Med. Assoc.*, **250,** 615
59. Harris, H. and Warren, F. L. (1953). Quantitative studies on the urinary cystine in patients with cystine stone formation and in their relatives. *Ann. Eugen*, **18,** 125
60. Rosenberg, L. E., Downing, S., Durant, J. L. and Segal, S. (1966). Cystinuria: biochemical evidence of three genetically distinct diseases. *J. Clin. Invest.*, **45,** 365
61. Scriver, C. R., Clow, C. L., Reade, T. M., Goodyer, P., Aurals Blais, C., Giguere, R. and Lemieux, B. (1985). Ontogeny modifies manifestations of cystinuria genes: Implications for counselling. *J. Paediatr.*, **106,** 411
62. Resnick, M. I., Goodman, H. O. and Boyce, W. H. (1979). Heterozygous cystinuria and calcium oxalate urolithiasis. *J. Urol.*, **129,** 52
63. Carpenter, P. J., Kurth, K. H., Blom, W. and Huijaamns, J. G. M. (1983). Heterozygous cystinuria and calcium oxalate urolithiasis. *J. Urol.*, **130,** 302
64. Brodehl, J., Gellissen, K. and Kowalewski, S. (1967). Isolated cystinuria in a family. *Klin. Wochen.*, **45,** 38

INDEX

absorptive hypercalciuria 40–1, 43, 45–6
acetazolamide 80
acid–base status 4, 37–8
acidification of urine 63
acidosis
  hyperchloraemic 4
  metabolic, calcium excretion in 37–8
acromegaly, calcium balance in 19–20
Addison's disease, hypercalcaemia in 19
alkaline phosphatase (AP) serum levels 4–5
alkalinization of urine 61, 80
alkalosis, metabolic 4, 26, 37–8
allopurinol 54, 60, 68
aluminium-containing antacids 67
aluminium toxicity 28
amino acids, sulphur-containing 36
aminoaciduria 73
  dibasic, isolated 85
aminohydroxypropylidene diphosphonate (APD) 8
antacids 26, 67
antibiotic therapy 62
antimalarial drugs 21
arginine 73, 74
arteriosclerosis, relationship to renal stone disease 71
ascorbic acid therapy 63, 83

Bantus, renal stone disease in 70

berylliosis 22
bicarbonate, sodium 61, 80
bone
  metastatic disease 5–6, 15–16
  resorption, increased 10, 42
  subperiosteal erosions 5, 6
bran 49
Brand's test 78
breast carcinoma, hypercalcaemia in 15, 16
breast milk of cystinuric patients 77
bronchial carcinoma, squamous 15, 17

cadaverine, urinary levels 78
calcitonin therapy 8
calcium
  adsorption by urinary macromolecules 69
  dietary intake 34–6, 40, 48, 55, 64
  excretion 5, 34
    acid–base status and 37–8
    dietary effects 34–7
    in primary hyperparathyroidism (PHPT) 10, 11
    seasonal variations 38
    sodium excretion and 7, 37
    see also hypercalciuria
  intestinal absorption 33–4, 35, 40, 41, 50
  load testing 44–5
  normal physiology 33–4
  plasma levels 3–4
  urinary levels 38–9, 65–7

INDEX

calcium-containing stones 47, 63–70
  in cystinuria 85
  inhibition by citrate 50
  risk factors 59–60
  uric acid levels and 68
  urinary calcium levels and 65–7
  urinary macromolecules and 69–70
  urinary oxalates and 67–8
  urinary pH and 65
  urine volume and 64
  see also hypercalcaemia *and* hypercalciuria
candidiasis, systemic 22
captopril 82
carcinoma, hypercalcaemia associated with 15–18
cardiovascular disease, relationship to renal stone disease 70–1
cellulose phosphate, sodium 51, 53
cholestyramine 67
choline 83
chondroitin sulphate 69
coccidiomycosis 22
colloids, urinary, *see* macromolecules, urinary
conjunctival calcification 3
conscious state, changes in 3
constipation 3
copper deficiency 81
corneal calcification 3
corticosteroid therapy 9, 21, 22, 24–5
creatinine, urinary 65
crystallization inhibitors 64
CT scanning of parathyroid glands 13
cyclic AMP, nephrogenous (NcAMP) 5, 45
cystine 73, 74
  plasma levels 78
  stones 73–5, 78
cystinuria 73–85
  clinical features 75–7
  diagnosis 77–8
  genetic counselling 84–5
  isolated 85
  life expectancy 77
  medical management 78–83
  prevalence and incidence 75
  renal replacement therapy 83–4
  surgical treatment 83

dichloromethylene diphosphonate (Cl$_2$MDP) 8
diet
  in cystinuria 79
  effects on calcium excretion 34–7
  in hypercalciuria 48–9, 55
  in hyperoxaluria 67
  incidence of stone disease and 36, 71
  uric acid stones and 60
1,25-dihydroxycholecalciferol (1,25(OH)$_2$D)
  dietary calcium intake and 35–6
  in granulomatous diseases 20, 22
  in idiopathic hypercalciuria 41
  in malignancy-associated hypercalcaemia 16–17
  in primary hyperparathyroidism (PHPT) 10
diphosphonates 8–9, 27, 52
diuretics
  loop 7
  thiazide, *see* thiazide diuretics
drug therapy
  antihypercalcaemic 7–9
  in cystinuria 80–3
  in hypercalciuria 49–52
drug-induced hypercalcaemia 23–7

endocrine disorders, hypercalcaemia in 18–20
endocrine neoplasia, multiple (MEN), syndromes of 9–10, 20
eosinophilic granuloma 22
ethane hydroxydiphosphonate (EHDP) 8–9
extracorporeal lithotripsy 62, 83
eyes, changes in hypercalcaemia 3

fertility, in cystinuria 77
fibre, dietary 49
fluid intake
  calcium stone formation and 23, 47–8, 55, 63–4
  in cystinuria 79
  infected stone formation and 63
  uric acid stone formation and 61
fluids, intravenous infusion 6–7

genetic counselling in cystinuria 84–5

INDEX

glucose, calcium excretion and 37
glutamine, in cystinuria 79, 82
glutamyl transferase (GGT) serum levels 4–5
glycosaminoglycans 70
gout 60, 77
growth impairment 76

haemodialysis, aluminium toxicity in 28
hand X-rays 5, 6
hexuronic acid 69
histoplasmosis 22
hyaluronic acid 69
25-hydroxycholecalciferol (25(OH)D) toxicity 24–5
hypercalcaemia 1–29
  causes 2
  drug-induced 23–7
  endocrine causes 18–20
  familial hypocalciuric (FHH) 5, 13, 27
  in granulomatous diseases 20–2
  in immobilized patients 22–3
  investigations 3–6
  malignancy-associated 15–18
    incidence and epidemiology 15–16
    management 18
    pathogenesis 16–17
    presentation 17
  medical management 6–9
  presentation and clinical features 1–3
  in renal failure 28–9
  see also specific hypercalcaemic disorders
hypercalcaemic crisis 3
hypercalciuria 33–55
  absorptive 40–1, 43, 45–6
  acid–base status and 37–8
  in acromegaly 19–20
  classification 39–42
  complicating parenteral nutrition 27
  definition 38–9, 65–6
  diagnosis 42–7
  dietary 40, 44
  idiopathic 33, 39, 40–2, 59
    diagnosis of subtypes 44–7
  in immobilized patients 22–3

  in primary hyperparathyroidism (PHPT) 10
  renal 41, 43, 45–7
  resorptive 42, 43, 45–6
  in sarcoidosis 21
  seasonal factors 38
  secondary 39–40, 44
  treatment 47–55, 66–7
    dietary 48–9
    drugs 49–52
    fluid intake 47–8
    of subtypes 52–5
  see also calcium excretion
hyperchloraemic acidosis 4
hyperoxaluria 67–8
hyperparathyroidism, primary (PHPT) 9–15, 39–40, 41
  with intermittent hypercalcaemia 42
  investigations 5, 13–14, 47
  management 14–15
  pathogenesis 9–10
  presentation and clinical features 10–12
hyperparathyroidism, secondary 41
hyperparathyroidism, tertiary (THPT) 28–9
hypertension
  in cystinuria 76
  in primary hyperparathyroidism (PHPT) 12
hyperthyroidism (thyrotoxicosis), hypercalcaemia in 18–19
hyperuricaemia 77
hyperuricosuria 54, 60
hypokalaemia complicating thiazide therapy 50
hypophosphataemia 36–7, 41, 54

ileostomy patients, uric acid excretion in 60
immobilization 22–3
infected stones 60, 61–3

keratopathy, band 3

lithium therapy, hypercalcaemia in 25–6
lithotripsy, extracorporeal 62, 83
loop diuretics 7

INDEX

lymphomas, hypercalcaemia in 16
lysine 73, 74
lysinuria, isolated 85

macromolecules, urinary 61, 64, 68, 69–70
magnesium ammonium phosphate (infected) stones 60, 61–3
malabsorption
  of amino acids 73
  hyperoxaluria in 67
mental retardation in cystinuria 76–7
mercaptopropionylglycerine (MPG) 82
metabolic acidosis, calcium excretion in 37–8
metabolic alkalosis 4, 26, 37–8
methionine, dietary restriction 79
milk–alkali syndrome 26
mithramycin 8
mucopolysaccharides, urinary 61, 69–70
mucoproteins, urinary 69–70
multiple endocrine neoplasia (MEN) syndrome 9–10, 20
myeloma, hypercalcaemia in 15, 16, 17

naphthaline 83
nephrocalcinosis 21, 24
nephrolithiasis, *see* renal calculi
neurological defects in cystinuria 76–7
nucleic acid metabolism 60
nutrition, parenteral, hypercalcaemia complicating 27

oestrogen therapy 15
1,25(OH)$_2$D, *see* 1,25-dihydroxycholecalciferol
25(OH)D (25-hydroxycholecalciferol) toxicity 24–5
ornithine 73, 74
orthophosphate therapy 51–2, 54; *see also* phosphate
osteoporosis 12, 15
oxalates
  dietary 67
  urinary 67–8

Paget's disease 5, 23

parathyroid gland
  adenomas 9–10, 25–6
    localization 13–14
  carcinoma 10
  enlargement 28–9
parathyroid hormone (PTH) 34, 35
  plasma immunoreactive (iPTH) 4, 13–14
parathyroid hormone (PTH)-like activity 16–17, 20
parathyroidectomy 14, 29
parenteral nutrition, hypercalcaemia complicating 27
penicillamine 81
peptic ulceration in primary hyperparathyroidism (PHPT) 12
percutaneous stone extraction 62
pH, urinary, stone formation and 61, 65, 78, 80
phaeochromocytoma, hypercalcaemia in 20
phosphate
  dietary intake 36–7, 65
  intravenous therapy 7–8
  oral therapy 9, 14–15, 51–2, 54
  renal tubular reabsorption (TmPO$_4$) 5
plasmin 69
potassium citrate 50, 61
protein, dietary 36, 40, 49, 79
PTH, *see* parathyroid hormone
purines, dietary intake 60
putrescine, urinary levels 78
pyridoxine 68, 81

radiology 5–6
radionuclide bone scanning 5–6
recurrent renal calculi 59–71
rehydration therapy 6–7
renal calculi
  calcium-containing, *see* calcium-containing stones
  cystine 73–5, 78; *see also* cystinuria
  environmental factors 70–1
  infected 60, 61–3
  recurrent 59–71
  removal techniques 62, 83
  uric acid 60–1

renal failure
  in cystinuria 83–4
  hypercalcaemia in 28–9
  in vitamin D intoxication 24
renal hypercalciuria 41, 43, 45–7
renal transplantation
  in cystinuria 83–4
  hypercalcaemia in 29
renal tubular acidosis, calcium excretion in 37–8
renal tubules, calcium excretion 33–4, 41
resorptive hypercalciuria 42, 43, 45–6

saline infusions 7
sarcoidosis, hypercalcaemia in 20–1, 41
sodium
  calcium excretion and 7, 37
  dietary restriction 48, 79
sodium bicarbonate 61, 80
sodium cellulose phosphate 51, 53
'stone clinic effect' 64, 66, 67, 68
struvite (infected) stones 60, 61–3
subperiosteal bone erosions 5, 6
sulphadryl therapy 80–2
sunlight, influence on calcium excretion 38

Tamm–Horsfall mucoprotein 68, 69
thiazide diuretics
  hypercalcaemia induced by 25
  in hypercalciuria 49–50, 52–4, 66–7
  potassium supplements 50, 54
thyroid–parathyroid subtraction scan 13
thyrotoxicosis, hypercalcaemia in 18–19
tuberculosis, hypercalcaemia in 21–2

ulceration, peptic, in primary hyperparathyroidism (PHPT) 12
ultrasound scanning of parathyroid glands 13
uric acid
  in calcium stones 68
  excretion 68
  stones 60–1
urinary tract infections
  in cystinuria 76
  stone formation in 61–3
urinary tract obstruction 63
urine
  acidification 63
  alkalinization 61, 80
  pH, stone formation and 61, 65, 78, 80
  volume 47, 48, 61, 64
urolithiasis, see renal calculi
uromucoid (Tamm–Horsfall mucoprotein) 68, 69

vegetarians 36, 49
vitamin A
  therapy 83
  toxicity 26
vitamin D
  intoxication 23–5, 41
  metabolism in granulomatous diseases 20–1, 21, 22
  status in primary hyperparathyroidism (PHPT) 10
  see also 1,25-dihydroxycholecalciferol

zinc metabolism 76
Zollinger–Ellison syndrome 12